THE COMPLETE
BOOK OF FOALING

THE COMPLETE BOOK OF FOALING

An Illustrated Guide for the
Foaling Attendant

Karen E. N. Hayes, D.V.M., M.S.

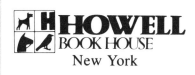

HOWELL
BOOK HOUSE
New York

To Dan: my love, my teacher
and my partner in learning

Howell Book House

Published by Wiley Publishing, Inc., New York, NY

For general information on our other products and services or to obtain technical support please contact our Customer Care Department within the U.S. at 800-762-2974, outside the U.S. at 317-572-3993 or fax 317-572-4002.

Wiley also publishes its books in a variety of electronic formats. Some content that appears in print may not be available in electronic books.

Library of Congress Cataloging-in-Publication Data:
Hayes, Karen E. N.
The Complete book of foaling: an illustrated guide for the foaling attendant / Karen E.N. Hayes.
p.   cm.
Includes index.
ISBN 0-87605-951-5
1. Horses—Parturition—Handbooks, manuals, etc.   2. Veterinary obstetrics—Handbooks, manuals, etc.   I. Title.
SF291.H36   1992
636.1'08984—dc20   92-18754   CIP

Manufactured in the United States of America.

20 19 18 17 16 15 14 13 12

BOOK DESIGN—DIANE STEVENSON/SNAP • HAUS GRAPHICS

CONTENTS

INTRODUCTION

There is a "scary" component to the birth process in horses—a lot of things *can* go wrong, and when they *do*, they do it in a big way, dramatically, with no apparent regard for the tenuous hold the new baby has on life. It is a powerful, dramatic and potentially violent event. Even though most foalings occur successfully without external assistance, the birth of a foal is potentially dangerous for both mare and foal because it is such a paradox of powers—a David and Goliath story. The mare is the powerful one, concentrating every ounce of her considerable strength into thrusting her foal out. The foal is dependent, vulnerable and fragile, subjected to the incredible forces of maternal labor, rapidly and forcibly squeezed through a narrow and unyielding passageway.

The foal is expected not only to survive the ordeal but also to make a rapid and essential adaptation from life *in utero*, where everything is done for him, to life outside the uterus, where he must quickly and efficiently learn to function independently. For example:

• Even though his lungs are fully developed at birth, they contain fluid that must be expelled, while an intricate sequence of chemical, neurological and muscular events must proceed without fail to dilate the nostrils, move the muscular diaphragm,

> **A**nything that acts to intensify the stresses of birthing will act against the foal's ability to adapt and survive the first moments of independent life.

expand the thoracic (chest) cavity and fill the bellows-like alveoli of the lungs with their first oxygen-rich air.

• In spite of the fact that the foal's heart has been beating since the earliest stages of the pregnancy, it has not been pumping any blood to his lungs, since the mare has been providing him with oxygen from her own lungs. In fact, the flow of blood through the fetal heart is essentially detoured to bypass his lungs, which, immersed in a "soup" of nourishing liquid, would be incapable of functioning properly at this stage—so strategically placed openings in the interior walls of his heart allow blood to whoosh through in the "wrong" direction until birth. At birth, the "holes" in the baby's heart must close, sealing off the interior chambers sufficiently to allow the foal's heartbeat to switch the direction of flow.

> The best way to prepare for attending an abnormal foaling is to understand, inside and out, what makes a normal foaling normal.

The adaptive process is crucial, and unless the foal is able, efficiently and accurately, to take over the processes that heretofore were performed by his dam, he will perish. A large portion of the foal's ability to make the transition from dependent life in the uterus to relatively independent life outside is directly related to what happens during the birthing process. Anything that acts to intensify the stresses of birthing will act against the foal's ability to adapt and survive the first moments of independent life. It is a difficult transition in any case, and any abnormalities or mishaps during parturition can lead to an overwhelming accumulation of physical stresses. After enduring eleven long months of gestation, the death of a long-awaited foal can be devastating. In most cases it is unnecessary and completely avoidable.

Preparing for a foaling is a lot like preparing for an IQ test in the sense that studying the night before the test would be unlikely to improve your score. The best way to perform well on an IQ test is to acquire, over an extended period of time, the broadest possible wealth of general knowledge so that each problem can be approached with confidence, logic and reasoning. The same is true of attending a foaling. It is highly unlikely that you could study enough about foaling *problems* to be able to handle emergency foaling situations optimally. Each individual foaling is unique, and any variation from the normal in position, condition, environment or history of the mare and/or emerging foal can make the recommendations for a particular type of dystocia (foaling problem) obsolete, insufficient and even injurious. Therefore, the best way to prepare for attending an abnormal foaling is to understand, inside and out, what makes a normal foaling *normal*. If every step of the normal foaling process is understood completely, then the foaling attendant will be better equipped to recognize early in the game when something goes wrong. The key to successful management of foaling problems is early detection and early correction.

Why is the birthing process in horses so violent? In nature, the predominant defense against predators appears to play a major role in determining whether the birthing process of a species is prolonged and relaxed or abbreviated and violent. Wolves, wild cats and other carnivores, for example (as well as their domestic counterparts), have essentially no worries about predators, and it may take many hours to deliver an entire litter. The fact that the bitch (female dog) or queen (female cat) has no plans to leave the birthing spot anytime soon is illustrated by the fact that she builds a nest some days before the event, and by the fact that her newborns are blind and unable to walk or run.

In contrast, the main defense horses have against predators is the ability to beat a hasty retreat. Horses would never build a "nest," since such an establishment would soon take on the distinct scent of "horse" and act as an advertisement to potential predators. This is especially true of the birthing spot—the fluids and membranes of foaling have a strong, distinctive odor which spells "easy meal" to the passing carnivore. Horses are, by nature, "fraidy cats"—they rely heavily upon their ability to outrun their enemies, and they identify all unfamiliar shapes and sounds as enemies until proven otherwise. They are reluctant to let down their guard and increase their vulnerability by lying down, a reluctance that was evolutionarily accommodated by stay-apparatus ligaments in their legs that allow them to sleep while standing. Mares in the process of foaling are completely incapacitated and vulnerable to attack by predators. It stands to reason that the mare's safety would best be served by getting the foaling process over with as quickly as possible so that she can get back to her feet and direct her attention once again to watching the bushes for real or imagined enemies. As a result, the birth process in horses is a powerful and rapid one.

> Horses would never build a "nest," since such an establishment would soon take on the distinct scent of "horse" and act as an advertisement to potential predators.

To compound the problem, the foal's main defense in life is to keep up with mama, and to that effect he is equipped with extremely long legs and a deep chest full of lungs. Combine these factors with the fact that the mare's physique, which is designed for speed, gives her a narrow pelvis, and the potential for problems should become clear.

Almost every mishap in the foaling process is something that can be prevented or corrected. With very few exceptions, foaling disasters that result in severe injury or loss of life are errors of nature that could have been dealt with successfully if a knowledgeable person had been present. Once in a while something will go wrong that is not correctable, no matter who is present, how much help is available and how much experience and expertise are at hand. But for the most part, there is no good reason that a foal should not be born with life and limb intact, and the foaling attendant holds the key to ensuring that nothing goes wrong.

With very few exceptions, foaling disasters that result in severe injury or loss of life are errors of nature that could have been dealt with successfully if a knowledgeable person had been present.

Follow along, then, this odyssey of the normal foaling, from the earliest pre-labor changes to the moment when the foaling process is completed. We will examine what is happening out of view inside the mare so that you can interpret the external events that can be observed. The foaling process should cease to be a mysterious event over which you have no control, during which you cross your fingers and hope for the best. You will learn when and how to intervene and when to refrain from intervening. As you become more and more comfortable with the normal situation, you will naturally become better qualified to recognize the abnormal, and you will be your own best insurance that mare and foal will survive and thrive.

CHAPTER 1

BEING THERE

No matter how knowledgeable you are about attending a foaling, none of your expertise will help if you aren't there to apply it. The most important aspect of helping your mare is *being there*, and it takes a certain amount of skill, forethought, arithmetic, persistence and good old-fashioned horsemanship to ensure that you are there when the time comes.

Section 1.1
The Arithmetic

Most textbooks state confidently that the length of gestation in the horse is 340 days. This should be used as a guideline only, since there is an extremely wide berth of variation from mare to mare and from one pregnancy to another. Some breeds of horse tend to carry their foals longer than others. Arabian horses of Egyptian lineage, for example, have been known to carry their pregnancies for an average of only 330 days, and this veterinarian has delivered normal, healthy Egyptian Arabian foals at 306 and even 304 days often enough as to consider it rather routine. By the same token, there are plenty of Egyptian Arabian mares that carry past the 340th day.

Contrary to previously published accounts and old wives' tales, ("she's overdue—it must be a stud colt"), there appears to be no statistically significant correlation between the sex of the foal and the length of the pregnancy. Furthermore, the previous history of a given mare ("she has always carried her foals for 338 days") does not necessarily indicate that forthcoming pregnancies will follow the same course. The only generalization that appears to hold up to long-term scrutiny is that the foalings that are due early in the foaling season (January through April) tend to go longer (340 days and beyond) than foalings that are due in the later, warmer months of the season. Research has shown that increasing the length of daylight with artificial lighting during pregnancy will cause mares to foal earlier than mares exposed to natural ambient light, suggesting that the timing of parturition is subject to the same sort of controls as is the onset of the breeding season. **The bottom line, then, is that your due dates should be expressed in terms of a 55-day range**, from about Day 310 to Day 365 from conception or last breeding date ("she's due between March 6 and May 1") rather than as the specific Day 340 date ("she's due April 4"), since the mare foals in response to foal readiness rather than to the numbers on a calendar. Based on this author's experience, **the foaling attendant must consider anything after Day 300 of pregnancy to be "fair game."** This is not to say that you must begin staying up all night with the mare once she passes her 300th day of pregnancy. This *is* to say, however, that no later than the 300th day, you should begin making specific observations and become acutely aware of certain clues that help narrow down the foaling date and make an intelligent decision about when to start spending nights in the barn. Additionally, if your mare's vulva has been sutured by a Caslick's procedure, she should definitely be opened up no later than Day 300 (see page 29).

The only sure thing about determining when a mare will foal is that you can never be absolutely sure until the foaling is over. However, there are several clues that the mare may give you, and in the majority of cases the clues will not mislead you. Taken individually, no single clue is strong enough or consistent enough to predict foaling time reliably. But when all available clues are observed and considered together, accurate prediction of foaling time is almost always assured.

Section 1.2
Shape Changes

The shape of the mare's belly, also known as the "way she's carrying," is often one of the first indicators of impending foaling. Earlier in the pregnancy the bulk of the pregnant abdomen's size tends to show up as fullness in the flank area and increasing overall width. As foaling time approaches, however, specific muscle groups in the floor and walls of the mare's abdomen begin to relax, and the shape and width of the pregnancy begin to gravitate downward, making the mare's abdomen seem to grow downward at its lowest point. A similar change takes place in women, and it is referred to in the same way: "The baby has dropped." As a general rule in horses this change in muscle tone distribution occurs during the last two to three weeks of pregnancy, so it isn't a fine-tuned indicator of impending foaling but is rather an announcement that the time is drawing near. Get into the habit of observing the mare's shape or silhouette from the front, the back and both sides. Although it's more obvious in mares that have already had a foal or two, you'll notice the change in shape in maiden mares as well. You simply have to look for it.

As the time of foaling nears, the mare's body begins to prepare itself by relaxing specific ligaments in the pelvic area. Relaxation of the pelvic ligaments becomes noticeable from the outside as a hollow or depression in the croup muscles. This is slightly more subtle than the abdominal shape change, but when the croup is observed from several angles, the looseness of the ligaments begins to show, just as the roof of a loosely staked tent begins to sag in the middle.

Section 1.3
The Milk

During the last weeks of pregnancy, most mares will begin to "fill" their udder or "bag up." Before udder development, the udder is collapsed, deflated in appearance and is carried up close

FIGURE 1.01
When viewed from the side, the silhouette of this mare at Day 320 appears thickened in the flank but the underside is still drawn up and tight.

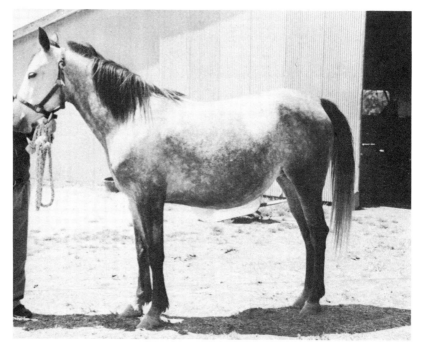

FIGURE 1.02
From the rear, notice how the bulk of this Day 320 pregnant abdomen's size is carried laterally, creating an ever-increasing width.

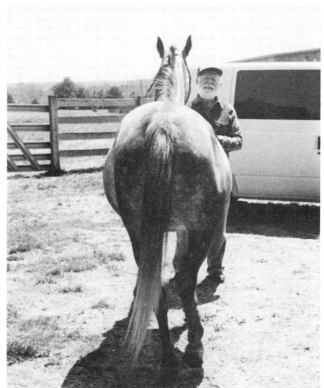

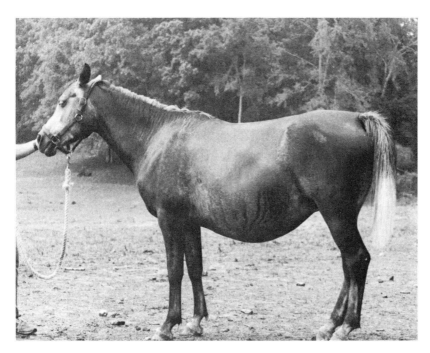

FIGURE 1.03
Day 332. Note the dropped abdominal silhouette of this mare that delivered four days after this photo was taken. The difference can be subtle, but with practice it becomes easier to see.

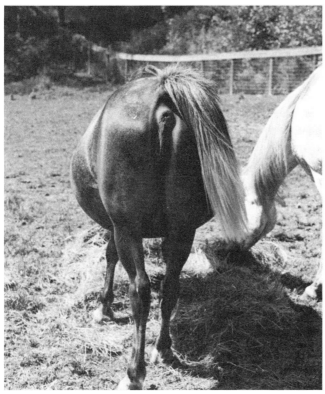

FIGURE 1.04
Same day as in photo above. Note the lowering of the abdominal width.

FIGURE 1.05 A, B, & C The relaxation of the pelvic ligaments is readily observable as a hollow or depression in the croup region. Each mare foaled within two weeks after the photo was taken.

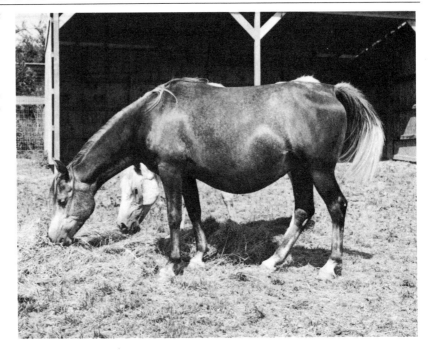

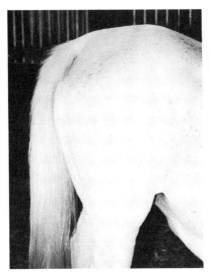

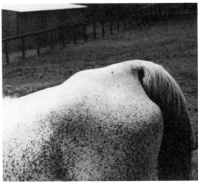

to the abdomen. As the pregnancy approaches its natural end, the matrix or framework of ducts and supporting structures within the udder begins to grow in anticipation of increased glandular volume that will be necessary to produce milk for the foal. Contrary to popular belief, the enlarging udder is not filling up with milk—it is enlarging due to an expanding milk "factory." After the supporting inner matrix of the udder is completed, the milk-producing glands begin to grow, and the udder and teats begin to take on an inflated, full appearance. At this point, the glands are secreting a substance, but it isn't technically milk yet. Some mares will bag up weeks before they foal, and other mares foal with what looks like very little bag. Some situations prevent normal udder development, and these will be discussed later. In the normal situation, however, **one of the most important determinants in predicting foaling time is the character of the liquid being produced in the udder**.

Your task at this time, then, is to express a drop or two of the udder's contents into your hand and examine it for characteristics that can be helpful in formulating your prediction. It is important that you work with your mare in this regard ahead of time so that she is accustomed to having her udder touched and handled. If you are thoughtful and considerate in your approach, you will meet with much less resistance.

MILKING SAFETY

The position of the mare's udder and the height of the average adult human make it awkward for a person to see, reach and manipulate the teats without getting into a dangerously vulnerable position. Just about everybody knows that the worst place to be when a horse kicks is behind the horse. What many people don't realize is that some horses can "cow-kick," a maneuver whereby the hind limb is brought forcibly forward and to the outside in a circular fashion, making it dangerous for a handler to stand anywhere within the radius of that kick. As this veterinarian can attest from personal experience, an accomplished cow-kicking mare can do serious damage to the person standing at her shoulder.

Mares that have never been known to behave in an aggressive manner around people may be pushed to the limit in the periparturient period (the period of time just before, during and just after foaling), and if ever a mare is tempted to cow-kick, it's while someone is messing with her sore udder right after she has foaled. This is especially true if she's irritable from abdominal cramps and not particularly happy with having to share her limited domain with foal and people. In fact, the mare that has never given her owners reason to expect aggressive behavior may be seen as more dangerous than the known kicker, since people will tend to be more trusting and careless around her.

One very valuable and relevant morsel you may have taken with you from high school physics class is the following formula:

$$Force = Mass \times Acceleration$$

Loosely translated in the context of a kicking mare, this means that the force exerted upon your body by a flying hoof will equal the mass (weight) of the hoof times the rate at which the leg is accelerating the hoof through the air. Since the kicking hoof accelerates (speeds up) until the leg is extended to complete the kick, the force of the kick will be highest at that point, which means that the worst place to stand would be about a leg's length away from the mare. By the same token, the best place to stand (if you *must* be kicked) is as close to the leg as possible, before it manages to achieve maximum acceleration, so that the force of the kick will be minimized. Furthermore, if you stand very close to the leg, the motion of the leg as it readies to kick is likely to shove you out of the way, and the mass of your body will help to stifle the force of the kick by preventing acceleration of the leg.

The most common approach to the mare's udder is also the most dangerous one. Most people stand at the mare's shoulder facing her hindquarters, bending over at the waist, crouching down slightly, reaching up to the udder. If a mare cow-kicks while you are in this position, your face will be at the point of maximum kick force. A safer approach would be to stand at the mare's flank or thigh, facing the udder, as close to her body as possible without being awkward. Keep one forearm or elbow pressed against the mare's hind limb, preferably in front of her stifle, if possible, so that any movement of that limb will be detected immediately and will be protected against by your arm. Resist the temptation to hunker down completely or kneel while manipulating the udder, since you will not be as capable of evasive action if the need should arise. Instead, stand with your legs slightly scissored apart, one ahead and one behind you, with both knees slightly bent. If possible, try to do your milking by feel rather than with visual guidance, since it is always preferable

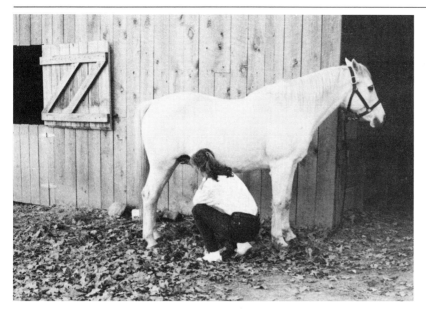

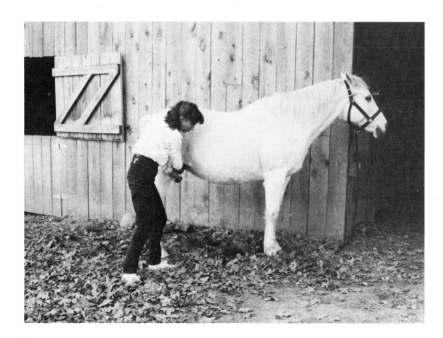

FIGURE 1.06 A, B
The person who approaches the udder from a position at the shoulder is at risk of being cow-kicked in the face. A better approach is to stand at the mare's flank or thigh, facing forward, as illustrated in Figure b. Once the mare has relaxed, the operator can move slightly forward if necessary, but contact should always be maintained with the hind limb in order to minimize kick force.

to keep your face and head out of the line of fire. Some operators find it helpful to press their head gently into the mare's flank while milking her.

Start by stroking the mare on her favorite itchy spot (most likely around the withers), and gradually, by stroking in a circular pattern, spiral your hand down along her belly until you are just in front of her udder. If it takes several minutes to gain her trust and work your hand down to the region of the udder, realize that the more you perform this exercise the easier it will become. If the mare is nervous and resentful and threatens to kick, it may be wise to stop here and start again later, each time going a little further. By the time you reach the ventral surface of her belly, she should be relaxed about your touch, and your hands should be warm. Now move your relaxed, open hand onto her udder (not the teat or nipple) and gently and shallowly massage the bag itself. As the mare learns that you aren't just going to grab her nipple or be thoughtlessly rough with her swollen and tender udder, she will relax and even begin to enjoy your gentle touch. Mares are often itchy in the area between the two halves of the udder and between the udder and the inner surface of the thighs, and you may be able to take advantage of the situation by gently satisfying the itch and demonstrating that your touch is a pleasure.

When you are certain that she has relaxed, gently move your hand so that you are holding one of the nipples at its base (where it attaches to the udder). Your hand should be in a flat pinching position, the way you would arrange it if you were going to make a shadow puppet on the wall. With your thumb and forefinger at the top of the nipple and your remaining fingers parallel to your forefinger, gently push your hand upward, giving the udder a gentle nudge. This will encourage some of the udder's secretions into the little reservoir (teat cistern) at the top of the nipple. Pinch, gently but firmly, the top of the nipple between your thumb and forefinger so that the liquid which is now in the teat cistern is trapped in the nipple and can't go back up into the udder, and with your remaining fingers moving serially, push the liquid down toward the tip of the nipple and out onto your waiting palm. Some people prefer to slip their thumb and forefinger down and off the nipple, as if whittling the nipple, but this is much more likely to irritate the mare, since the friction of thumb and forefinger repeatedly rubbing down along the nipple will eventually lead to chafing. People who use this method often moisten their fingers with their own saliva in order to reduce the friction on the nipple, but this is very bad technique, since human saliva is teeming with bacteria. The nipples should not be a place for the new-born foal to become ill!

The best way to practice the proper milking technique is to poke a pinhole into the tip of one finger of a physician's latex examination glove. Pour half a cup or so of water into the glove and, hanging it from one hand over the sink, practice "milking" it with your other hand, remembering that you don't want to rub the nipple—you want to pinch it at the top with your thumb and forefinger to keep the water from spurting back into the hand of the glove, and then, with your thumb and forefinger still holding that pinch, work the water down to the tip and out the hole with your remaining three fingers.

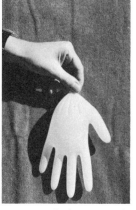

FIGURE 1.07
A latex examination glove filled with water makes a good model for practicing proper milking technique.

The time to start checking the secretions of the mare's udder is when the udder and nipples begin to look inflated. If you find that the mare is relatively relaxed about having her udder handled, but you have a very difficult time expressing any fluid, it's probably too early and you can wait for a day or two before trying to milk her again.

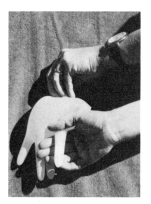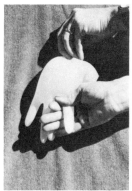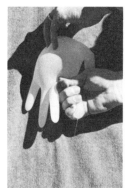

FIGURE 1.08 A, B, & C
a. Nudge the bag upward gently to fill the "teat cistern,"
b. pinch off the "nipple" at its base and
c. squeeze serially downward, forcing the "milk" out.

As a rule, as the mare gets closer to foaling, it becomes easier and easier to express fluid from the udder, and the character of the fluid progresses from

1. clear and watery, to
2. thin but cloudy, to

3. yellow-tinged and increasing in viscosity, like floor wax, to
4. definitely amber-colored and syrupy-thick, to
5. skim milk, to
6. opaque white milk.

As the character of the "milk" secretions changes along the progressive six steps from clear and watery to opaque white, the frequency of your examinations should increase accordingly, from every other day, to once a day, to at least twice a day by the time it has reached character #3. Sometimes the character of the fluid progresses so rapidly that your observations may miss a step. In many cases the latter changes occur during the late afternoon and early evening hours of the day, and it is not uncommon for a mare's secretions to be amber-colored syrup one moment and opaque white milk an hour later.

At the risk of oversimplifying, the calcium content of the mare's milk plays a major role in determining whether or not the milk is white. The more calcium it contains, the more opaque white it will be. This is the basis for the "new" foaling predictor test strips that have recently become available on the market. The strips, which were originally developed to measure "hardness" (mineral content) of tap water, also can be used to estimate the calcium content of the mare's udder secretions. Since the calcium content in the milk is directly proportional to the whiteness of the milk, it is really rather redundant to use test strips on milk that is obviously changing color and character in ways that easily can be observed with your eyes. Nevertheless, if you need the additional security of an "official" test, the foaling predictor test strips are a relatively inexpensive and accurate investment to add to your predictive tools.

In many cases, just before the fluid begins to take on a milky white appearance, you may find flecks of white or yellowish solid material suspended within the clearer fluid. This may be the result of calcium that has precipitated out of solution due to its rapidly increasing concentration. As the milk changes in composition to accommodate the rising calcium levels, the flecks dissolve and are incorporated into the whitening solution.

Interestingly, the hormone oxytocin, which causes the uterine contractions of hard labor, also causes "milk letdown," the phenomenon whereby milk streams out of the udder with minimal coaxing. Research has shown that oxytocin is less effective in both of these functions if the circulating calcium level in the bloodstream is low. Calcium is stored in the body in the bones, and the level of calcium that is permitted to circulate in the blood is regulated by the parathyroid glands, small bean-shaped glands located adjacent to the thyroid gland in the neck. It is likely that the change in character of the mare's udder secretions, indicating an increasing concentration of calcium in the bloodstream, is evidence that the parathyroid glands are preparing the mare for an impending surge of oxytocin by allowing a higher level of calcium in the circulation. It is well known that calcium levels in the mare's bloodstream increase dramatically prior to foaling, and simply taking the time to check the character of the mare's milk is a quick and relatively accurate way of monitoring this calcium increase.

By the time the secretions of the udder have become yellowish and viscous, the remaining steps can occur quite rapidly. Even though most mares do not foal until their milk has become opaque white, it is not uncommon for a mare to begin the foaling process at the yellowish syrup stage of udder secretion, and by the time the foal has been delivered, the milk has become opaque white. Furthermore, in some cases, the milk remains yellowish syrup for up to 24 hours after the foal has been born. It is advised, therefore, that your all-night vigils begin no later than the point when the mare's udder secretions are yellowish and thickened.

Most horse breeders know that as a mare approaches foaling, the teats of her developing udder begin to accumulate "beads" or plugs of colostrum at their tips. These beads are actually dried wads of the viscous, syrup-like secretions that leak out in an insignificant

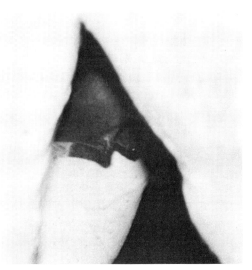

FIGURE 1.09
Beads of colostrum accumulated at the tips of the teats

amount as the udder develops. Many horsemen believe that these dried secretions help to plug up the teat and prevent valuable colostrum from leaking out onto the ground before the foal is born. They shudder at the suggestion that you would disturb these plugs by expressing a drop or two of milk into your hand every day to check its character, because they believe that by disturbing the plugs, you're allowing the udder to leak colostrum later. This is simply not true. Milk will not stream out of the udder until it is signaled to do so by the hormone oxytocin. The plugs at the ends of the teats occur as innocently as the dried secretions that accumulate each night in the corners of your eyes. They serve no function—they're simply there.

The biggest mistake that can be made in assessing a mare's readiness to foal is to fail to look for the clues. Bear in mind that some mares can "build a bag" and begin to ooze colostrum practically overnight. The fact that she had absolutely no bag last night is not reason enough to skip your examination this morning! Remember also that there are some conditions that can *interfere* with the development of a mare's udder and/or the manufacture and letdown of milk. For example, there is evidence to suggest that certain individuals are genetically or otherwise unable to create or maintain the hormonal "cocktail" needed to make milk—interestingly, many of these mares are also "silent heat" mares, meaning that they are seldom or never receptive to a stallion, even when they have a large, breedable follicle on their ovary. In most cases, however, mares that fail to produce milk are victims of some external problem—such as when their nutritional status is inadequate (too little calcium, perhaps, or too little protein), or if their general health is in question. Recent research has suggested that obese mares produce less milk than mares that are slightly underweight. And there is the infamous problem of fescue grass poisoning—certain types of fescue pasture and hay are susceptible to contamination by a fungus that virtually shuts off the mare's mammary glands. Mares that fall victim to fescue syndrome are likely to carry their pregnancies longer than usual, and they may have absolutely no udder development at all when the foal is finally delivered.

Section 1.4
Vulvar Changes

A significant but less reliable clue to impending parturition is the change in color of the mucus membranes (the inside) of the mare's vulva. The theory is that as foaling draws nearer, there is an increase in circulation to the pelvic area of the mare, and this increase in circulation is visible as hyperemia (a deepening of the pink color) of the vulvar mucosa. This can be misleading, because any physiological event that alters the circulation in the pelvic area, even to the slightest degree, can change the color of the vulvar mucosa. Straining to defecate, posturing to urinate, and even the forces of gravity, such as when a mare is grazing uphill so that her rear end is lower than her front end, or when a mare is lying down for a nap, can make the vulvar mucosa appear pinker. When a mare lies down at night to sleep, the mucosa of her vulva becomes almost scarlet in color, but this is simply a function of her position and does not necessarily indicate that parturition is imminent. This is not to say that you should not check the vulvar mucosa for change in color; the message here is to check the vulva, but consider your observations in conjunction with the whole picture.

Another significant but less reliable clue is the degree of relaxation of the vulva. Ordinarily, the vulva, which is a vertical slit with somewhat thick lips, has a certain degree of muscle tone. Under various circumstances, including imminent foaling, the musculature of the vulva relaxes, the length of the slit increases, and the entire vulvar structure appears flabbier and less of a barrier than usual. One experienced horseman describes the vulva in this state as resembling the end of an "old empty coat sleeve." Once again, this can be misleading, because various external influences can make the vulva more or less relaxed. The sleeping mare, for example, is in a general state of relaxation, and the tone of the vulva is appropriately reduced. Furthermore, when a mare is lying down, there is increased pressure on her abdomen by the hard surface of the ground, and this increased pressure will cause her anus, vulva and the perineum (the surface between the anus and vulva) to pouch outwardly to a certain extent. The result can be a vulva that is not only partially open

15

and relaxed in appearance, but it may also be partially everted, so that the first inch or two of the vulvar mucosa (insides) is actually visible. This is often mistaken as an indication that the mare is starting to foal.

Additionally, a mare may voluntarily tighten up her vulva in certain situations, and if you happen to look at her vulva during this time, you may be misled into thinking that the pelvic muscles have not yet begun to relax. For example, most mares will wink their vulvar/clitoral area after urinating, which makes the vulvar lips appear less relaxed. Some mares will tighten up their vulvar area if you touch them around the tail or buttocks or if they anticipate that you are about to touch them in that region. Some mares will tighten up if you simply walk around to the rear. It is important, therefore, that you make your observation quietly and without prior warning, preferably without touching the mare. For the same reason, it's best to make this observation before opening the vulva to check for mucosal color.

But there's a better reason to check the vulva. During pregnancy, the closed cervix is sealed with a mucus plug that is thick, tacky and the color of rose quartz. When foaling is imminent, the relaxing cervix begins to release its grasp on the plug, and portions of the waxy plug begin to fall into the vagina and out the vulva. This is called the "bloody show." When you see this, there's little doubt that foaling will take place within 24 to 48 hours. But to see it, you have to look!

Section 1.5
Rectal Temperature

Recently it has been reported that the mare's body temperature will change prior to foaling, and recent research has confirmed that the temperature change, although relatively small, is significant enough to be a very useful predictor. Although additional work in this area is needed, at this point it appears that the extra time and effort required to measure and keep track of the mare's temperature is quite worthwhile. Earlier researchers had reported that the mare does not show a significant temperature change prior to foaling, but these studies had been done with the old-fashioned standard mercury thermometers. With highly accurate electronic thermometers now readily available and relatively inexpensive, the apparent changes in body temperature prior to foaling are now simple to detect.

As is true in many mammalian species, the mare's body temperature fluctuates normally throughout the day. The fluctuation is somewhat consistent, however, in the sense that the body temperature at a specific hour of a given day will be about the same as the body temperature at that same hour on other days. This is called diurnal rhythm. As a general rule, the mare's body temperature in the late afternoon will be higher than in the morning, and in order to use the change in temperature as a predictor of impending foaling, the normal daily temperature fluctuations in each individual broodmare must be determined ahead of time. At least seven days' measurements should be obtained as a baseline before any variation in temperature should be interpreted as significant.

Beginning at Day 300, and using an electronic digital readout thermometer, the mare's rectal temperature is taken at the same hour every morning (choose a time between 7 A.M. and 8 A.M. and stick to it) and every afternoon (choose a time between 4 P.M. and 5 P.M. and stick to it). The exact temperature reading is recorded on a chart. The temperature readings should remain relatively constant for each time frame in spite of changes in the weather; i.e., the morning rectal temperatures should be about the same each morning and the afternoon rectal temperatures, although generally higher than the morning readings, will also remain about the same each afternoon. The temperature reading may be elevated if the mare is ill or has recently exercised or otherwise undergone physical exertion prior to taking the measurement, so it is important to keep some external factors as consistent as possible. Bear in mind that in order to generate an accurate reading, the tip of the thermometer must be in contact with the rectum itself, not in the space of the rectal lumen—if the mare's rectum is "ballooned" with gas at the moment you take the temperature, you may get an unusually low reading. To avoid this, develop a routine that works for you—lubricate the tip, insert it gently the same distance every time, then angle it so the tip rests against the ceiling of the rectum. And use a thermometer that "beeps" when ready to read.

FIGURE 1.10
Sample temperature chart on a mare that foaled thirty hours after the low temperature reading was taken. Note that the morning temperature on the day of the foaling had returned to normal, which often (but not always) happens. This should demonstrate how important it is not to miss a scheduled measurement, since the temperature drop would have been missed if the 5 P.M. reading on 2/23/90 had not been taken.

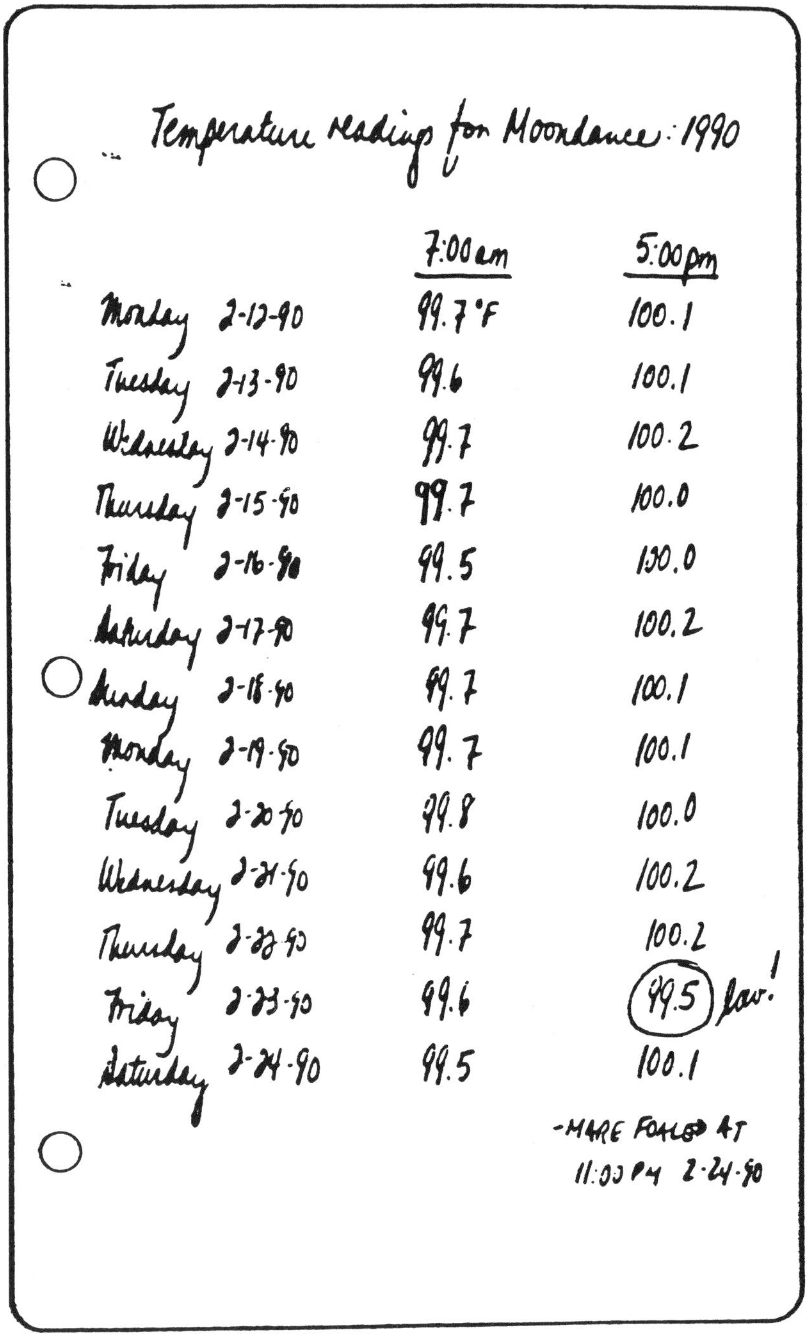

Temperature readings for Moondance: 1990

		7:00 am	5:00 pm
Monday	2-12-90	99.7 °F	100.1
Tuesday	2-13-90	99.6	100.1
Wednesday	2-14-90	99.7	100.2
Thursday	2-15-90	99.7	100.0
Friday	2-16-90	99.5	100.0
Saturday	2-17-90	99.7	100.2
Sunday	2-18-90	99.7	100.1
Monday	2-19-90	99.7	100.1
Tuesday	2-20-90	99.8	100.0
Wednesday	2-21-90	99.6	100.2
Thursday	2-22-90	99.7	100.2
Friday	2-23-90	99.6	(99.5) low!
Saturday	2-24-90	99.5	100.1

—MARE FOALED AT
11:00 PM 2-24-90

18

Within approximately 18 to 24 hours prior to foaling, the mare's body temperature at its regularly scheduled checking time should be lower than usual, and the difference may be as much as one whole degree (but usually it's only a little more than 0.5°F) lower than the usual reading. Remember that each clue should be considered in concert with the others; i.e., if the mare's milk is turning white but the temperature change has not occurred, **do not** ignore the milk and go to bed. By the same token, if the milk is still clear but the temperature reading is suddenly about 0.7° F lower than usual, **do not** ignore the temperature change and go to bed. Sometimes one clue is all you get—don't ignore it when it's given to you. And in the extreme case, if the mare is very close to the traditional due date of 340 days and has little or absolutely no udder development, and the temperature has dropped, **do not ignore the temperature drop!** Many factors can inhibit the normal development of the udder, and some mares will foal with absolutely no milk at all. Furthermore, when a mare foals without milk, there are usually other problems as well, and odds are increased that the foal will be at increased risk of injury or death due to oxygen deprivation at birth, so it is especially important that a knowledgeable attendant be present when the foal is born.

Section 1.6
Assorted Lesser Changes

Other less consistent changes occur in some mares and can contribute to your overall assessment of foaling time but should definitely not be relied upon alone. Some mares will exhibit an enlargement of the "milk vein" (the large blood vessel that runs just under the skin along the lower abdomen toward the udder on each side of the body) a day or two before foaling. Some mares exhibit varying degrees of swelling or edema in the lower portions of the legs and along the midline of the abdomen in front of the udder during the last few days of pregnancy. And some mares will refuse their grain during the last day or two before foaling. These are unreliable changes that probably indicate changes in circulation from the increasing weight of the

FIGURE 1.11
Ventral edema, seen most often in older mares, may be an indication of mild to moderate circulatory impairment.

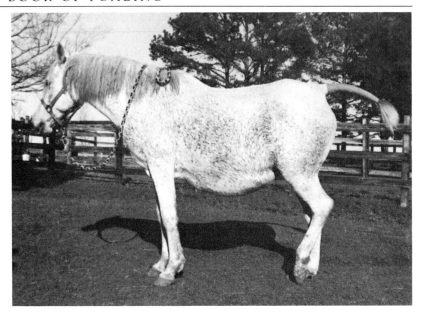

fetus, lessened activity on the part of the fatigued, burdened mare and decreased appetite from overall discomfort. They may be indicative of medical problems and should always be investigated by a veterinarian.

Section 1.7
Electronic Predictors

One additional type of tool that is available for predicting foaling time is the electronic surveillance device. The equine marketplace is full of gadgets and gizmos that are promoted as "foolproof" in getting you to the barn in time to see your foal born. Since the application of this technology in equine obstetrics is still relatively new, many of the systems are still in need of refinement. None should be relied upon entirely. But if you are in need of additional help in monitoring your mare and can afford the cost of such devices, following is a summary of the available types, their strengths and weaknesses.

1. Vaginal This system utilizes a small electronic device that is sutured to the vulva of the mare. When it is pushed out of position by the emerging foal, an alarm goes off. Foaling problems can get a head start with this design, as will become clear later in the section on Stage II labor, since the emerging of the foal marks the time when you should already be *finished* with several important pre-foaling tasks, such as checking the status of the foal's position and making any necessary corrections. By the time the delivery has gotten this far, any problems will have become well established and may be beyond repair.

2. Vertical/Horizontal   This system is based on the premise that if the mare lies down, flat out on her side, she's probably in labor. A transmitting device is attached in the vertical position on the side of the mare's halter. It becomes horizontal, of course, if the mare lies down in the "flat out" position with her head on the ground. This sets off the alarm. Unfortunately, there are many ways in which mares are able to set off the alarm when they aren't in labor, including scratching the sides of their heads on the top of the fence, reaching under a low barrier to grasp a mouthful of grass or spilled feed, and simply lying down for an innocent nap. Admittedly, mares in the last weeks of pregnancy are reluctant to lie out flat because breathing is difficult in this position when the weight and bulk of the heavily pregnant abdomen press into the chest, but they are also extremely fatigued and may try the position several times for short periods before finding it too uncomfortable to stay down. Hence the owner of a vertical/horizontal type foaling alarm may have several false alarms each night. After several nights of interrupted sleep, some weary individuals with understandably clouded judgment have actually turned off the alarm, gone back to sleep, and missed the whole thing. Some are designed to go off only when the horizontal position is maintained for over 10 seconds, eliminating many of the false alarms. However, once again, this system alerts the attendant after it's already too late for most foaling problems to be corrected easily. Furthermore, some (admittedly few, but some) mares will foal while standing, never tripping the alarm.

3. "Electric Eye"   This system, which will work only if the mare is in a stall, consists of beams of light that are interrupted when the mare is standing, but when the mare lies down, the beam of light emitted from one side of the stall is allowed to connect with a receptor on the other side, completing the circuit and setting off the alarm. The obvious shortcoming in this system is the myth that pregnant mares lie down only when in labor (but at least it won't set off the alarm when she's only scratching her head). Another shortcoming is the occasional mare that delivers her foal while standing.

4. Sweat Detector   This system is based on the premise that mares break into a sweat before going into full labor. The device, which is patterned after the skin temperature electrodes in lie detectors, sets off an alarm when the skin temperature rises past a preset level, just before sweating commences. Unfortunately, many mares achieve this temperature level at times other than during labor, and others seem to remain "cool as cucumbers" throughout the entire delivery. The system excels over many others, however, in the sense that it strives to detect Stage I of labor rather than Stage II, and when the alarm goes off there should be time for the foaling attendant to evaluate the situation and correct any problems.

5. Abdominal Press   This system was designed to measure changes in the diameter of the mare's abdominal girth, presuming that when the mare "bears down" to "push" during labor, her abdominal girth becomes larger. The mare wears a flexible surcingle that sets off an alarm when stretched. Urinating, defecating, coughing, sneezing, and lifting a hind limb to scratch an ear have all been known to set off the alarm. Furthermore, by the time the mare is in active labor, it may be too late to correct any problems.

6. Closed-Circuit Television Camera   Although no alarm system is connected with this system, it has the advantage of permitting close observation of the mare from a distance, avoiding unnecessarily disturbing her. It also permits the attendant to remain in comfortable quarters, regardless of the weather, until his/her presence in the barn is needed. It requires, of course, that the attendant remain awake and alert.

CHAPTER 2

THE BIRTH CANAL

The developing fetus spends the bulk of its life forward of the birth canal, in the abdomen of the mare. It isn't until labor actually begins that the birth canal is entered. That's the reason it's called the birth *canal*—it's a passageway through which the foal must go in order to exit the uterus. The reason the foal is not in the birth canal until then is because the birth canal is closed and functionally locked by barriers that form its boundaries.

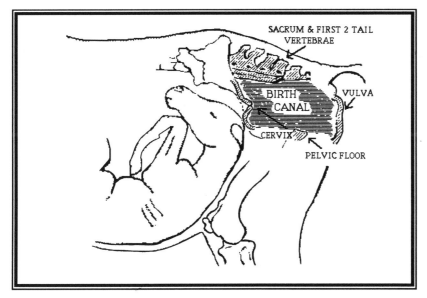

FIGURE 2.01
The fetus is "locked" out of the birth canal until delivery begins. The birth canal is defined by its six boundaries, which form its ceiling, its floor, and its anterior, posterior and side walls.

The anterior or forward barrier to the birth canal is the cervix. This is a muscular barrier, a tough, tubular, purse string–like passageway that is tightly contracted during pregnancy, forming a rather impressive blockade to all but the most vigorous intrusions. It isn't until the cervix softens, of its own volition in response to chemical signals, that actual labor begins.

FIGURE 2.02 A, B
Vaginal view (inset) and side view of cervix. The cervix is tightly closed (left) or loose and easily pushed open (right) in response to hormonal signals it receives from the mare.

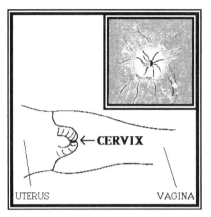
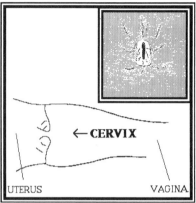

The posterior or rear boundary of the birth canal is the vulva. This too is a muscular boundary, its main function being to isolate the birth canal from outside contamination. In se-

FIGURE 2.03
A Caslick's closure involves cutting away the edge of the vulvar lips and suturing them together in order to improve the quality of the barrier between the vagina and the outside world.

lected cases, the upper two-thirds of the vulva can be surgically sutured closed by a procedure called a Caslick's closure. The rationale is to improve the barrier between the vagina and the outside world in cases where the vulva no longer provides a competent seal against contamination.

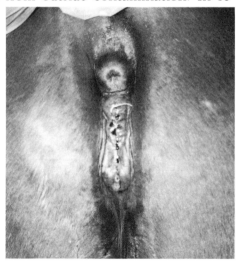

The salient point about the muscular cervix and vulva is that in the event of a foaling problem, these barriers are more likely to tear rather than to prohibit the foaling process. There

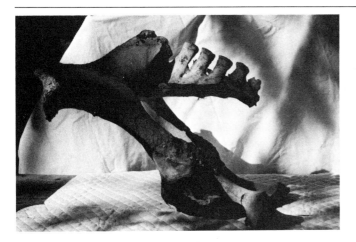

FIGURE 2.04
Side view of bony pelvis, sacrum and first coccygeal (tail) vertebrae of a Thoroughbred mare that stood 16 hands tall. These parts form the bony portion of the birth canal; the ceiling, floor and side walls.

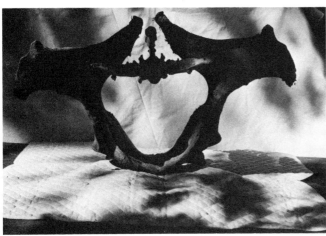

FIGURE 2.05
Same pelvis, showing the birth canal as it would appear to the foal on its way out.

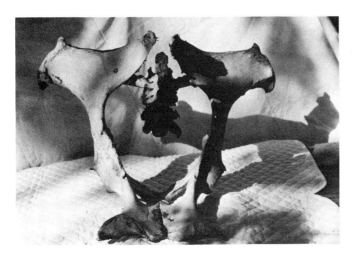

FIGURE 2.06
Same pelvis, showing the birth canal from the outside looking in. Note that the opening is smaller at the posterior aspect of the canal, making the canal cone-shaped.

are exceptions to this rule, but for the most part a problem at either of these locations would result in more damage to the mare than to the foal.

The same cannot be said for the remaining boundaries of the birth canal. The lateral walls, floor and ceiling are formed by the bony pelvis. The bony sacrum and first one or two coccygeal vertebrae (vertebrae of the mare's tail) are fused together to form the ceiling of the birth canal and, in turn, are fused as a unit to the bony pelvis. The result is a hard, unyielding, unforgiving passageway that does not stretch or expand to accommodate the foal. There is no room for error here, and it is this portion of the birth canal where the most potential for damage to the foal exists. Even the slightest mistake in the foal's position can result in a serious situation if that mistake is not corrected before the foal becomes dangerously wedged in the canal. Positional mistakes are best corrected before the foal enters the birth canal—early detection and early correction.

CHAPTER 3

PREPARATION

Section 3.1
Choosing a Veterinarian

Equine veterinary medicine is a specialty, and equine reproduction and obstetrics are even further specialized. It is highly recommended that a veterinarian who specializes in equine medicine, and preferably one who has an added interest in equine reproduction and obstetrics, attend to your breeding and foaling needs. It is essential that you choose a veterinarian who is willing and available to respond to after-hours emergency calls, since most mares foal between 10 P.M. and 6 A.M. It is advised to arrange to have a veterinarian who is experienced and interested in equine obstetrics on the premises while your mare is foaling, since problems will be much more serious if professional help is not provided immediately. In most cases, the foaling will be absolutely normal, and the veterinarian will have driven to the farm "for nothing," but when a problem does occur, the slightest delay in getting help can turn the problem into a life-threatening situation. Therefore, the veterinarian you choose should be one who is willing to attend all foalings, not only when a problem is already obvious. If your late-night foaling call is met with the response "Call me if there are any problems" instead of "I'm on the way," you probably should have chosen another veterinarian.

27

It is also important that you choose a veterinarian with a well-equipped mobile unit so that most of the specialized equipment that might be needed during a foaling problem would always be available in his or her vehicle. Ideally, the capability of administering emergency oxygen would be included in this specialized equipment. Try to choose a veterinarian who is organized, so that it is easy to find supplies and equipment in the mobile unit during an emergency. The days of the old country vet who carries only a bottle of "bute" and a stomach tube are over, and it is your responsibility to find and acquaint yourself with a veterinarian who is up to date and well equipped. By the same token, you should be willing and able to pay for this top-of-the-line service. Mares are pregnant for approximately eleven months—you should be able to accumulate an "emergency fund" during those eleven months to cover any expenses that might arise during the foaling.

Introduce yourself to the veterinarian of your choice long before the foaling date, and, if feasible, employ this veterinarian's services for your mare's routine care so her special characteristics and needs will be known and your late-night emergency foaling call will be met with some semblance of recognition and acceptance. Be sensitive to the fact that veterinarians work around the clock and have little time to themselves, and try to be as educated as you can about your horses and their needs so that you can be an asset to their care when the veterinarian is in attendance. Additionally, be prepared to receive instructions over the telephone for tasks that the veterinarian may want you to do with your mare while waiting for his or her arrival.

Keep your own organized records of the mare's breeding dates and the 55-day range of expected foaling time, and when the time for foaling approaches, take it upon yourself to call the veterinarian to give fair warning that the time is near and that a late-night call should be expected in the near future. Do not expect the veterinarian to keep records of your mare's foaling time, since he or she cannot assume that you will *want* his help unless you ask for it. And again, for reasons that should become clear later in this book, **do not wait until there is an obvious foaling problem to call the veterinarian**—by that time you are already in deep trouble. Ideally the veterinarian should be there when the foaling starts, and it is up to you to see the signs and make the call in time.

Section 3.2
Check Caslick's

No later than Day 300, every pregnant mare should be checked for previous Caslick's surgery. A Caslick's closure is an optional procedure whereby the upper portion of the mare's vulva is sutured (stitched) closed to prevent vaginal contamination and possible infection of the uterus. Some authors suggest opening the Caslick's closure only two weeks before the due date, but this will be too late for some mares, and the damage to the vulva can be extensive if a delivery rips through a closed Caslick's. The best method of opening a Caslick's is to have the veterinarian "numb" the vulva with a series of local anesthetic injections first, then cut on the "seamline" and treat the raw edges as an ordinary open wound. For more on this subject, see Stage I, Section 4.3.

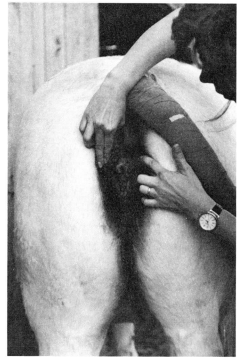

FIGURE 3.01
Natural, unsutured vulva

Section 3.3
Prefoaling Vaccines

Four to six weeks prior to the Day 340 "due date," all pregnant mares should be given a "booster" inoculation with a good-quality "four-way" vaccine (Eastern and Western equine encephalomyelitis, tetanus toxoid, and influenza). Be sure that the vaccine is approved for use in pregnant mares. This booster should increase the quality of the mare's colostrum and provide improved protection for the newborn against those diseases. Optimal immune response to vaccination requires from two to three weeks, so vaccinations given too close to foaling will not have time to stimulate an immune response, preventing the beneficial effect on the colostrum. Conversely, many practitioners believe that the stress associated with vaccination can lead to premature delivery or abortion. Since foal survival is unlikely in premature deliveries prior to Day 300 of pregnancy, it is unwise to vaccinate any *earlier* than Day 300 in case it plays a role in causing the mare to deliver early. The decision to give multiple vaccines should be made with special consideration and care for the same reason.

Nevertheless, if a particular disease is endemic in your area, if an outbreak of a particular disease is suspected or if your horses and/or premises have been exposed to a particular disease, additional vaccines for your mare and her colostrum may be warranted. Examples of some of these diseases are leptospirosis (for which no equine vaccine is currently available), *Streptococcus equi* ("strangles"), rabies, and Potomac horse fever. Boosters for equine rhinopneumonitis ("rhino") should be done earlier in the pregnancy, at the fifth month, the seventh month and the ninth month.

Section 3.4
Nutrition

The best way to provide proper nutrition in horses has always been controversial, partly because there are different schools of thought on what horses require to be healthy, and partly because the quality and availability of feedstuffs vary widely according to location. The situation is made more complex by the fact that each individual horse has its own unique way of handling its feed, activity level and the stresses and demands of life. Furthermore, in spite of the fact that there are many talented and knowledgeable horsemen in this world, the percentage of individuals possessing a real understanding of the basic facts of nutrition is very small compared to the percentage of individuals with opinions about nutrition and no real knowledge to back them up. As a result, people who really have no idea what they're doing are formulating and altering diets for horses and may unknowingly be contributing to reproductive, performance and general health problems.

The fact that horses need free access to clean, fresh water is not controversial. All horses should be able to drink freely at all times unless they have just been exercised or are otherwise overheated. The average horse in the average circumstance drinks 10 to 15 gallons of water per day, so provisions should be made to supply each horse with free access to at least 30 gallons per day, since variation in weather, ambient moisture and activity levels will vary the water requirements. The fact that the water must be fresh and clean can't be stressed enough. Some horses will refuse to drink water, even when they are thirsty, if the water is scummy or off-smelling. If hay or other feed material is spilled into the water, particularly during warm weather, the water can quickly become quite soured. Some horses have the nasty habit of passing manure into their water tubs, which is more likely to be an accident of circumstance rather than a purposeful act, and no horse will drink manure-contaminated water. Algae growth in water tubs can be another serious health risk, particularly in warmer climates. Large clean rocks stacked in the water tub against one end will provide a means of escape for thirsty bugs, squirrels, raccoons, and other critters that may otherwise drown in the tub and further foul the water. Obviously in very cold weather the water source may freeze, and horses are not able to eat enough ice or snow to satisfy their water needs, nor are they inclined to try. Electric heaters for stock tanks can be dangerous if improperly installed (i.e., not grounded properly) or if even slightly damaged, and the resultant shock to the thirsty horse can easily be fatal.

Automatic watering devices can eliminate the water contamination problem, since their water receptacles are relatively small and are automatically refilled often. A significant problem with automatic waterers, however, is that they tend to foster a false sense of security about the water supply, making it seem unnecessary to check if the horses have adequate fresh water. If a plumbing problem renders the automatic waterers nonfunctional and the horse's caretaker fails to check the water source regularly, the horses may already be suffering from dehydration before the plumbing problem is discovered. Furthermore, the use of automatic waterers makes it impossible to assess the volume of water each horse drinks, which may be important in certain circumstances when water intake information is needed. Whatever watering system is used, the people responsible for the horses' well-being should be certain that clean, fresh water is always available.

TABLES 3.1 & 3.2
Daily intake recommendations are always changing as research continues and our knowledge of nutrient requirements grows. Each individual horse will have specific needs that vary from the "official" recommendations because of individual differences in digestion, metabolism, overall health, demeanor, environmental stresses and other factors. Nonetheless, many horses that receive "nothing but the best" from their owners are fed diets that are severely unbalanced with respect to general needs. The figures in tables like these should be used as guidelines when formulating equine diets.

TABLE 3.1   NRC RECOMMENDATIONS FOR D.E. (DIGESTIBLE ENERGY) AND PROTEIN INTAKE IN A HORSE EXPECTED TO WEIGH 400KG (880 LB) WHEN MATURE

	D.E. in MCal/KG	PROTEIN
Weanling	13.03	14.5%
Yearling	13.80	12.0%
2-Year-Old	13.89	9.0%
Mature Working Horse	variable	7.7%
Mature Maintenance	13.86	7.7%
Last 90 Days Pregnancy	15.52	10.0%
1st 3 Months Lactation	23.36	12.5%
Later Lactation	20.20	11.0%

TABLE 3.2   NRC RECOMMENDATIONS FOR CALCIUM & PHOSPHORUS DAILY INTAKE IN A HORSE EXPECTED TO WEIGH 400KG (880 LB) WHEN MATURE

	CALCIUM (GRAMS)	PHOSPHORUS (GRAMS)
Foal to 6 months	33	20
Weanling	34	25
Yearling	31	22
2-Year-Old	25	17
1st 8 Mo. Pregnancy	23	14
Last 3 Mo. Pregnancy	34	23
1st 3 Mo. Lactation	34	23
Later Lactation	50	34
Mature Maintenance	23	14

Too often the equine diet is designed with *human* likes, habits and tastes in mind. Horses were designed to eat a high-fiber, relatively poor quality diet in small, constant doses rather than in two or three large meals the way humans eat. In the natural non-pregnant situation, horses spend roughly 50 to 60 percent of a 24-hour period eating (grazing), and each feeding bout lasts from 30 minutes to 4 hours, depending on the palatability of the feed and the degree of hunger at the initiation of feeding. Compare this to the way most horses live today, confined to a stall and fed at the whim of their human caretakers, often given a diet that may require less than an hour or so of total eating time. Mares that are heavily pregnant have shorter eating spells, since they have less room in their abdomens for feed. Consequently, they need to have the opportunity to eat more often.

Many body systems cooperate to help digest the feed, and one important factor is the digestive fluid bile. Bile is a digestive liquid that is manufactured in the liver at a constant rate, whether the animal is eating or not, and in most mammalian species, the constant trickle of fresh bile is shunted into a muscular storage sack (the gall bladder) until needed. Shortly after a large meal is ingested, the gall bladder squeezes and empties its accumulated bile onto the passing slurry of recently eaten food and contributes to the digestive process. Obviously this system was designed for animals like humans that eat large, separate meals. The horse has no gall bladder, since it was designed to eat constantly rather than in large meals—in horses, the constant trickle of fresh bile spills directly into the duodenum (first part of the small intestine) rather than detouring into a storage sack, since there is supposed to be a fresh supply of feed going through the duodenum almost constantly. As a result, horses that are fed meals once or twice a day are at increased risk of poor digestion, malnutrition and colic, despite the fact that their feed may be an expensive "top of the line" product. Their well-meaning owners would be better advised to spend their money on a good-quality balanced vitamin/mineral supplement and clean free-choice grass hay or grass pasture access.

This is especially true for the pregnant mare, because in addition to creating increased nutritional demands, the rapidly growing pregnancy also takes up more and more space in the abdomen, crowding the digestive system and making it even

33

TABLE 3.3   CALCIUM AND PHOSPHORUS CONTENT OF SOME COMMON FEEDS

	CALCIUM	PHOSPHORUS
Alfalfa Hay	1.30%	0.25%
Bermuda Hay	0.35%	0.31%
Barley	0.05%	0.37%
Oats	0.07%	0.37%
Soybean Meal	0.31%	0.70%
Wheat Bran	0.12%	1.43%
Bone Meal	0.71%	0.46%
Limestone	0.67%	0.00%
Calcium Carbonate	0.34%	0.00%

TABLES 3.3 & 3.4
To be used as guidelines only. For accurate calculation of any individual horse diet, the actual feeds used must be analyzed for their nutrient content (or, in commercially packaged feeds, read the nutrient breakdown on the package).

TABLE 3.4   SELECTED NUTRIENT CONTENT OF SOME COMMON GRAIN PRODUCTS AND CONCENTRATES

	good OATS	poor OATS	shelled CORN	hulled BARLEY	MANNA ELITE*	corn OIL	CALF* MANNA	wheat BRAN	soybean MEAL
PROTEIN (%)	13.0	11.0	9.0	11.0	14.0	0	25.0	15.0	45.0
D.E. (Mcal/kg)	3.0	2.4	3.5	3.2	2.90	8.5	0	2.8	3.2
FIBER (%)	10.0	13.0	2.0	6.0	7.5	0	6	10	6
CALCIUM (%)	0.1	0.09	0.02	0.08	0.75	0	1.0	0.1	0.25
PHOSPHORUS (%)	0.35	0.30	0.31	0.40	0.50	0	0.6	1.2	0.6
FAT (%)	7.0	6.6	3.9	2.0	8.0	100	0	4.6	0.9

* Manna-Pro Corporation

more difficult to accommodate the large volume of separate meals. To make matters worse, the meal-fed mare gets so hungry between meals that she is more likely to eat too much too fast at mealtimes, overwhelming the digestive enzyme systems. As a result, much of the meal is inadequately digested by the time it reaches the large fermentation vat called the cecum, and excessive gas production can result. The equine digestive system was designed to accommodate and move a certain volume of gas, but when the volume of gas is excessive and the available space in the abdomen is decreased due to a rapidly growing fetus, serious problems can occur. As a result, in addition to providing a diet that fails to meet the pregnant mare's needs, the well meaning but uninformed horse owner may actually be harming the mare by setting her up for colic and other health problems.

CALCIUM

During the last trimester of pregnancy the mare will require more calcium. This is an extremely important mineral for many essential functions, including milk production, bone formation in the developing baby and muscle contractions during labor. The amount of calcium fed must be considered in concert with the amount of phosphorus in the diet, since the body always considers these minerals together and the equine system prefers that they be provided in the ratio of approximately 1.5 calcium to 1.0 phosphorus. If the diet fed is exceptionally high in phosphorus, the calcium requirement increases in order to maintain the proper ratio. Unfortunately, most of the commonly fed equine feeds are naturally high in phosphorus and low in calcium. Grass hays and most commonly fed grains (oats, barley, corn) are very high in phosphorus and low in calcium, making the calcium requirement higher in order to establish the proper ratio of calcium to phosphorus. Legume hays, especially alfalfa, are generally a good source of dietary calcium, and the pregnant mare will benefit from a carefully meted ration of alfalfa hay added to her predominantly grass hay diet. The proportion of alfalfa hay needed will depend on the content of the grass hay already being fed, but some equine pathology experts have attributed many problems to diets which contain too much alfalfa, so it is important to add only enough alfalfa to meet the calcium requirements and keep the primary emphasis in the diet on the grass hay. For help in calculating a proper ration, see pages 40–45.

If alfalfa hay is not available, extra calcium can be provided in several forms. The least expensive source of calcium is the ground limestone product calcium carbonate, available in most feed stores in 50-pound bags. A measuring tablespoon of calcium carbonate contains about 10 grams of dietary calcium. The pregnant mare in the last trimester of pregnancy needs about 30 to 40 grams of calcium per day (the requirement increases as the foaling date approaches), so her needs should be met by giving 3 tablespoons of calcium carbonate a day and increasing it to 4 tablespoons by the beginning of the final 30 days of the pregnancy.

There are some problems with this method, however. First, calcium carbonate tends to settle at the bottom of the feed tub when mixed with dry grains such as oats or barley, and since it tastes like chalk, most mares will not make an effort to clean it up. Adding a small amount of water or molasses to the grain ration will help keep the calcium carbonate from settling out. However, once the problem of getting the calcium into the mare's mouth has been solved, another problem arises. Calcium ingested in this form is not well absorbed into the mare's bloodstream, and much of what is eaten is simply passed out in the manure. Nutritionists have discovered that many dietary minerals are readily absorbed when chemically "linked" to a substance that the body absorbs more easily. A few commercially available mineral supplements are prepared by this process (called chelation), which links the minerals to albumin, a high-grade protein. The body readily recognizes and absorbs the albumin, and the calcium that is chelated to it "piggybacks" a ride into the bloodstream. These products are expensive, but the calcium is highly biologically available and virtually none is wasted.

The percentage of mares that successfully complete the foaling process with an inadequate foundation of dietary calcium is testimony to the fact that the body is remarkably able to adapt and make excuses for its deficiencies. At some point, however, the debt can become overwhelming, and the mare is forced to walk a thin line between "barely getting by" and falling apart. The health of the developing fetus hangs in the balance.

The ideal solution to the problem of maintaining the proper calcium-phosphorus balance in the pregnant mare is to provide a diet that contains the highest possible quality of calcium so that the absorbed components are determinable. In other words, if the diet contains the proper proportion of calcium and phosphorus, but much of the calcium passes through without being absorbed because it is not a chelated product, it is impossible to assess the resulting deficiency since you don't really know how much (if any) was absorbed and how much passed through in the manure. **Overdosing on calcium is as injurious as the deficiency state,** and making the necessary corrections requires that you know the current levels being absorbed. When good alfalfa or high-quality chelated mineral supplements are used, the amount of calcium *fed* is roughly equal to the amount *absorbed,* and providing the proper amount is a matter of simple arithmetic (see pages 42–43).

PROTEIN

As a general rule, total protein intake in the nonpregnant mare and during the first two-thirds of pregnancy should be between 10 percent and 11 percent. This is roughly the protein content of most good-quality grass hays, so maintenance of most non-pregnant mares usually does not require the addition of grain products, with the possible exception of some Thoroughbred mares. However, most people do feed some grain to their horses anyway, and as long as the quality is good and the quantity is not excessive, no harm is done. The rule of thumb for nonpregnant mares is to feed a quantity of grain that is approximately 0.5 percent of the mare's weight. In other words, if the mare weighs approximately 900 pounds,

$$900 \text{ lb} \times 0.005 = 4.5 \text{ lb of grain per day}$$

her total daily grain ration should not exceed 4.5 pounds per day. (If a mare is already overweight, even half this amount would be too much.) Of course, the quality and digestibility of grain products can vary widely, and the safest way to assure that the horse is not harmed by the protein content of a grain product fed is to **never feed your mare a grain product that contains more than 14 percent protein.** Furthermore, the actual diet formulation should be done with careful calculation using the product's analysis, as described in detail on pages 40–45, rather than using the thumbnail formula above. Excessive protein fed during pregnancy is believed to stress the mare and can produce excess ammonia (by-product of protein metabolism), which can cross the placenta and interfere with normal neurological development of the fetus. It also places an increased burden on the mare's kidneys. Therefore, it is extremely important not to overdo it on the protein.

Protein requirements during the last trimester of pregnancy are increased over what is required in the nonpregnant state. As the protein requirements increase, the addition of a calculated amount of a good-quality grain product is needed to boost the protein content of the overall diet to 12.5 percent. The increase should be done gradually, following approximately the formulas below:

> **Month 8 of pregnancy: Increase grain to 0.5% body weight + ½ lb *for 900-lb mare*: = 4.5 lb grain + 0.5 lb = 5.0 lb grain per day.**
>
> **Month 9 of pregnancy: Increase grain to 0.5% body weight + 1 lb *for 900-lb mare*: = 4.5 lb grain + 1 lb = 5.5 lb grain per day.**
>
> **Month 10 of pregnancy: Increase grain to 0.5% body weight + 1.5 lb *for 900-lb mare*: = 4.5 lb grain + 1.5 lb = 6.0 lb grain per day.**
>
> **Month 11 of pregnancy: Increase grain to 0.5% body weight + 2 lb *for 900-lb mare*: = 4.5 lb grain + 2 lb = 6.5 lb grain per day.**

Even if all the nutrition the mare needs is supplied in her grain, she still needs hay for the fiber.

These formulas are intended as approximations only, and they are meant for horses being given free-choice, high-quality grass hay in concert with the grain. Note that the calculated amounts of grain recommended are total daily intake, not the amount to be given at each meal. It is astounding how many horse owners give their horses 5 or 6 pounds of grain two or three times each day—these horses are a ticking time bomb, teetering on the edge of laminitis (founder), kidney failure, colic and/or a variety of other serious problems.

Again, the quantity of grain needed will depend on the quantity and content of the hay being fed, and the only way to know what's in the hay is to have it analyzed. Most agricultural and veterinary laboratories routinely do feed analyses, and it is a good idea to submit samples of your feed on a regular basis so that any adjustments that are necessary can be made in your horse's overall diet.

CARBOHYDRATES

Carbohydrate requirements in horses vary widely with the physical demands placed on them. For the purposes of this book, **the most important thing to remember about carbohydrates is that they are potentially dangerous in horses**. Very few equine diets are deficient in carbohydrates. The majority of equine diets contain excessive carbohydrates. The equine digestive system is extremely sensitive to excessive carbohydrates, and a diet that contains an overdose of carbohydrate can actually be fatal. Therefore, when calculating a ration for a pregnant mare, particularly when calculating how much grain should be fed in order to meet the protein requirements, the carbohydrate content of that diet should be calculated primarily to determine whether or not *too much* carbohydrate is being fed.

FIBER

The amount of hay a horse eats is important from the standpoint of digestive tract functioning as well as nutrient requirements. Even if all the nutrition the mare needs is supplied in her grain, she still needs hay for the fiber. Otherwise she is at increased risk of colic. Most nutritionists recommend that the average horse receive about 1 to 2 percent of her body weight a day in grass hay. (If your horse is fortunate enough to have access to good-quality grass pasture, the best rule of thumb for calculating the quantity eaten is that a growing pasture provides approximately 2 pounds of grass per hour of grazing.) As her pregnancy grows and takes up space in the abdomen, the mare's ability to accommodate large volumes of high-fiber feed becomes increasingly impaired, so she may choose to eat less hay at any one feeding. Nevertheless, it should be available to her at all times so that she can nibble small amounts of hay more frequently, since her total daily hay requirement will remain the same. If good-quality grass pasture is available, much of the fiber requirements can be met by grazing. Remember, however, that it is the fiber content of the hay, not the moisture content, that helps keep things moving in the digestive tract. The lush, green, juicy grass that grows in the spring is most likely to lead to intestinal impaction, since it is so low in fiber, and this catastrophe is best avoided by providing the usual ration of hay to the pastured mare. Most mares will "sense" their fiber need and will spend quite a bit of time eating the dry hay, even when the juicy green grass appears so much more appetizing.

Measurements and Ration Calculation

Most people report the diets they feed to their horses in terms of "scoops" or "coffee cans." In order to calculate the diet, these measurements must be converted into pounds or kilograms. Remember that a 3-pound coffee can may hold 3 pounds of *coffee*, but the amount of *grain* it holds may be more or less than 3 pounds. The weight of hay is also very difficult to estimate, and when asked how many pounds of hay their horse gets, most people get a blank look and mumble something about "flakes" or "sections." When finally induced to buy or borrow a scale to weigh their horse feed, most people are surprised at how off-target their rations are.

In order to calculate the nutrient content of your mare's overall diet, you will have to gather all the information you can on the content of each ingredient. Most commercially mixed horse feeds have protein content (expressed as %) and carbohydrate content (expressed as DE, or digestible energy, in units of megacalories) listed on the package. If not, contact a reputable agricultural laboratory and arrange to send a sample of your feed for analysis. A sample of your hay should also be sent, and the proper method of obtaining a good representative sample will be outlined by the laboratory director. The hay sample submitted should include a portion of several randomly selected bales rather than just one bale, since the quality of hay may vary from bale to bale.

For the limited purposes of this discussion, simply find the protein content, digestible energy (DE), calcium and phosphorus in each component of the diet. If your horse's diet consists of several different products such as hay, grains and supplements, be sure to find the protein, DE, calcium and phosphorus content of *each* of the components.

Let's say that a mare is in her first trimester of pregnancy, and she weighs 850 pounds. If a large animal scale is not available to determine exact weight, her weight can be estimated using a girth tape (available at most tack shops, feed stores and through horse-supply catalogs). The mare's current diet consists of the following:

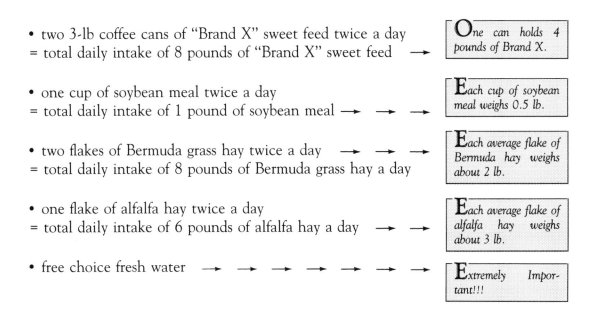

- two 3-lb coffee cans of "Brand X" sweet feed twice a day
= total daily intake of 8 pounds of "Brand X" sweet feed →

*O*ne can holds 4 pounds of Brand X.

- one cup of soybean meal twice a day
= total daily intake of 1 pound of soybean meal → → →

*E*ach cup of soybean meal weighs 0.5 lb.

- two flakes of Bermuda grass hay twice a day → → →
= total daily intake of 8 pounds of Bermuda grass hay a day

*E*ach average flake of Bermuda hay weighs about 2 lb.

- one flake of alfalfa hay twice a day
= total daily intake of 6 pounds of alfalfa hay a day → →

*E*ach average flake of alfalfa hay weighs about 3 lb.

- free choice fresh water → → → → → → →

*E*xtremely Important!!!

- We know from the Brand X bag that the product is **14% protein** and has a **DE of 3 Mcal/kg.**, and it contains **.08% calcium** and **0.40% phosphorus.**
- The soybean meal package lists its **protein content** as **45%** and its **DE** as **3.2 Mcal/kg**. It contains **0.31% calcium** and **0.70% phosphorus.**

• The lab analysis of the grass hay showed that it contains **10% protein** and **1.7 Mcal/kg.** It contains **0.35% calcium and 0.31% phosphorus.**

• The lab analysis of the alfalfa hay showed that it contains **14% protein** and has a **DE of 2.04 Mcal/kg.** It contains **1.30% calcium** and **0.25% phosphorus.**

So, first we calculate the protein in the diet:

8 lb sweetfeed × 0.14	=	1.12 lb protein
1 lb soybean meal × 0.45	=	0.45 lb protein
8 lb grass hay × 0.10	=	0.8 lb protein
6 lb alfalfa × 0.14	=	0.84 lb protein
23 lb feed		3.21 lb protein

So the mare is getting:
3.21 ÷ 23 =
0.14 or 14% protein.

Next we calculate the calcium and phosphorus in the diet:

8 lb sweet feed × 0.0008	=	0.01 lb calcium
1 lb soybean meal × 0.0031	=	0.0031 lb calcium
8 lb grass hay × 0.0035	=	0.03 lb calcium
+6 lb alfalfa × .0130	=	0.08 lb calcium
23 lb feed		0.12 lb calcium

There are 454 grams in a pound, so this mare is getting:
454 × .12 =
54.48 grams of calcium

8 lb sweet feed × .0040	=	0.03 lb phosphorus
1 lb soybean meal × .0070	=	0.007 lb phosphorus
8 lb grass hay × .0031	=	0.02 lb phosphorus
6 lb alfalfa × .0025	=	0.02 lb phosphorus
23 lb feed		0.08 lb phosphorus

There are 454 grams in a pound, so this mare is getting: 454 × .08 =
36.32 grams of phosphorus

so:

The ratio of calcium to phosphorus in this diet is 54.48 to 36.32
= $\boxed{1.5 \text{ to } 1}$

Finally, let's calculate the carbohydrate (DE) content of this diet. In order to do this, we must convert the measurements of each feed component from pounds to kilograms. There are about 2.2 pounds in each kilogram, so the diet contains:

8 lb ÷ 2.2 = 3.64 kilograms (kg) sweet feed
1 lb ÷ 2.2 = 0.45 kg soybean meal
8 lb ÷ 2.2 = 3.64 kg grass hay
6 lb ÷ 2.2 = 2.73 kg alfalfa

And to calculate carbohydrates:

3.64 kg sweet feed × 3 Megacalories (Mcal)/kg	= 10.92 Mcal
0.45 kg soybean meal × 3.2 Mcal/kg	= 1.44 Mcal
3.64 kg grass hay × 1.7 Mcal/kg	= 6.19 Mcal
2.73 kg alfalfa × 2.04 Mcal/kg	= 5.57 Mcal
	24.12 Mcal

So, the diet this mare is receiving contains the following:

- 8 lb grass hay + 6 lb alfalfa hay
- 14% protein
- 54.48 grams of calcium and 36.32 grams of phosphorus for a calcium-to-phosphorus (Ca:P) ratio of 1.5 to 1
- 24.12 Mcal of digestible energy.

How does this compare to what she *should* be receiving?

• At 850 pounds, she should receive 1 to 2 percent of her correct (ideal) body weight per day of grass hay, which is 8.5 to 17 pounds of grass hay. This mare gets only 8 pounds of grass hay, which is not enough, but some of her fiber needs are being met by the alfalfa, so let's set this point aside for now.
• Her protein level should be between 10 percent and 11 percent. Her current diet is 14 percent protein, which is much too high. Remember that excessive protein can be potentially dangerous to the mare and her developing fetus.

• Her daily calcium intake should be about 30 grams per day, balanced with a phosphorus intake of 20 grams so that their ratio is 1.5 to 1. Her current diet contains over 54 grams of calcium and 36 grams of phosphorus. They are properly balanced, *but the amount of each component is too high.*

• Her daily DE should be about 14 Mcal per day, unless she is on a regular exercise schedule. Her current diet contains over 24 Mcal of digestible energy per day. This is extremely high for a relatively inactive mare. Remember that *excessive carbohydrate is extremely dangerous* to the mare, and this diet makes her a prime candidate for laminitis.

It should be clear at this point that the example diet in this exercise needs some adjusting. A good place to start would be to reduce the protein and carbohydrate levels. For example:

• Since soybean meal is high in both protein and in carbohydrates, and since the other components of this mare's diet are more than adequate in protein and carbohydrates, the soybean meal should be eliminated completely from this particular diet.

• Unless this mare is being exercised, the amount of sweetfeed should also be drastically cut to, for example, 2 pounds per day.

• Let's also reduce the amount of alfalfa hay she's getting to 3 pounds a day, since she needs more grass hay and her protein level is so high, and let's increase her grass hay to 12 pounds a day.

Now let's calculate this new diet:

PROTEIN:

1.90 ÷ 17 =

| 11.0% protein |

2 lb sweetfeed × 0.14	= 0.28 lb protein
12 lb grass hay × 0.10	= 1.20 lb protein
3 lb alfalfa × 0.14	= 0.42 lb protein
17 pounds of feed	1.90 lbs protein

CALCIUM & PHOSPHORUS:

2 lb sweetfeed × 0.0008 = 0.0016 lb calcium
12 lb grass hay × 0.0035 = 0.0420 lb calcium
3 lb alfalfa hay × 0.0130 = 0.0390 lb calcium
17 pounds of feed ———————— 0.0826 lb calcium

0.0826 lb at
454 grams/lb =
37.50 grams calcium

2 lb sweetfeed × 0.0040 = 0.0080 lb phosphorus
12 lb grass hay × 0.0031 = 0.0372 lb phosphorus
3 lb alfalfa hay × 0.0025 = 0.0075 lb phosphorus
17 pounds of feed ———————— 0.0527 lb phosphorus

0.0527 lb at
454 grams/lb =
23.93 grams phosphorus

The ratio of calcium to phosphorus in this diet is
37.50 to 23.93 = 1.57 to 1

DIGESTIBLE ENERGY (CARBOHYDRATE):

2 lb sweetfeed ÷ 2.2 = 0.91 kg.
0.91 kg × 3 Mcal/kg = 2.73 Mcal

2.73
9.27
+2.77
14.77 Mcal

12 lb grass hay ÷ 2.2 = 5.45 kg
5.45 kg × 1.7 Mcal/kg = 9.27 Mcal

3 lb alfalfa hay ÷ 2.2 = 1.36 kg
1.36 kg × 2.04 Mcal/kg = 2.77 Mcal

A summary of this amended diet shows that the mare is now getting:

• **12 pounds of grass hay** (well within the recommended range of 8.5 to 17 pounds)

• **11.0 percent protein** (10 to 11 percent is recommended, so we're right on target)

• **37.50 grams of calcium** and **23.93 grams phosphorus** for a ratio of **1.57 to 1** (close to our target of **1.50 to 1**)

• **14.7 Mcal of digestible energy** (pretty close to the recommended 14 Mcal)

45

The mare's requirements will change as she enters the third trimester of her pregnancy, foals, and begins to lactate, requiring up to 12.5 percent protein, 23 Mcal per day of digestible energy, and 50 grams of calcium balanced with 30 grams of phosphorus (see Tables 3.1 and 3.2). The original example diet which was too rich for the mare in the first trimester of pregnancy (8 pounds sweetfeed, 1 pound soybean meal, 8 pounds grass hay and 6 pounds alfalfa hay) may be quite suitable for the mare when she is lactating. As always, any changes in the diet should be made gradually so the mare's digestive system can adjust to them.

If the diet being fed is correct with respect to protein, carbohydrate, fiber and mineral requirements, but the mare is too thin or otherwise looks unhealthy, she should be examined by a veterinarian and evaluated for parasite load, dental problems and general health problems that can interfere with the normal digestion and absorption of nutrients. If the veterinary examination reveals no abnormalities except confirmation that the mare is too thin, it is possible that the fat content of the diet needs to be increased. Like humans, horses have different metabolic rates that make individuals more or less efficient in the way they burn their fuel.

The judicious addition of fat to a diet can be an extremely effective way to increase the energy component (calories) without increasing the potentially dangerous carbohydrate and protein levels. Research has shown that horses can tolerate surprisingly high levels of fat in their diets (up to 16 percent of the DE) with apparently none of the health risks that would accompany an increase in carbohydrate or protein levels. Most commercial equine diets contain only 2 to 6 percent fat, but the horse can utilize as much as 16 percent fat in the total ration without adverse affect. Furthermore, whereas 1 gram of carbohydrate provides 4 calories of energy and 1 gram of protein provides 4 calories of energy, a single gram of fat provides 9 calories of energy, making fat a much more efficient dietary calorie booster.

If evaluation of an underweight mare indicates that she simply needs more calories, favorable results can be obtained by carefully adding from 2 to 16 ounces of vegetable oil (such as corn oil) to her grain ration daily. The addition of any dietary component, including vegetable oil, should always be done gradually so that the horse's digestive system can acclimate, and the larger the volume of oil given each day, the more important it is to divide it into as many small portions as possible throughout the day. Higher levels are often accompanied by loose stools, so be on the lookout for signs that an oil-supplemented mare is getting too much oil. If it is determined that a mare needs as much as 16 ounces of oil per day, she should be started out with only 2 ounces a day, then increased by 0.5 ounce each day until, by the fourth week, the oil ration has reached 16 ounces per day. Again, if the individual's tolerance to oil has been exceeded, loose manure will result, and the oil ration should be reduced to a level well beneath that point. Visible results, both in terms of body fat and in terms of coat gloss, should take about six weeks to appear maximally.

The specific dietary needs of horses in general and of pregnant mares in particular are too complex to cover completely in the context of this book. As a general rule, however, the following basic concepts should be considered when feeding the pregnant mare:

1. Remember that all horses were designed to eat small amounts constantly of a diet characterized by high fiber and low palatability. If you must feed your mare in meals, divide her total daily intake into as many small meals as possible so that her hunger level never rises very high and so that her crowded digestive tract can enjoy a constant supply of a more manageable volume.

2. Make the main component of the diet a high-fiber grass hay, rather than a legume hay, since most legumes (such as alfalfa and clover hays) are very "rich" in protein and may stress the digestive and kidney (renal) systems of the mare and contribute to developmental problems in the fetus. Add grain products only as needed to supplement the protein and energy requirements as detailed in the previous section.

3. The best way to provide extra calcium to the pregnant mare is to give the proper amount of alfalfa (with its calcium content known from laboratory analysis) or to supplement the diet with a chelated calcium product. Whichever method is used, be sure to calculate how much is needed to provide the required calcium in proper balance with phosphorus. Re-

frain from giving more alfalfa than is needed, since excess protein can be harmful.

4. Become acquainted with the specific characteristics of the feed in your part of the country, especially with respect to the problems those characteristics may cause in your pregnant mare. If your area is reported to be deficient in the mineral selenium, for example, it may be necessary to supplement your mare's diet with this essential **but very toxic** mineral. If the mare needs selenium, supplementing her diet with selenium will help her in many ways, but if the mare receives more selenium than she needs, illness and even death can result. Therefore, have the feed and the mare's blood tested for selenium levels before making any attempt to supplement the diet with selenium.

5. Some areas actually contain too much selenium in the soil, and certain plants will contain the soil's high selenium content in their leaves and stems. This can pose a risk of selenium poisoning, making it necessary to provide a safer feed source. If your area is suspected of being too high in selenium, have your feed, pasture plants and your mare's blood tested for selenium content.

6. If your area has fescue grass in the pastures, and/or if the hay you provide contains fescue, there is an increased chance that the mare may fall victim to "fescue poisoning," a complex of disease conditions that can cause low fertility, abortions, weak foals, stillbirths, thick placentas and, most commonly, lack of milk production. The problem is not the fescue grass itself; the problem lies with a fungal agent that commonly "infects" fescue grass. If your hay or pasture contains fescue grass, contact an agriculture expert and arrange to have the pastures and hay tested for the fungus. If the pastures or hayfields are infested, there is currently no reliable way to eliminate it without destroying the grass and replanting. For this reason, it is best to avoid planting fungus-susceptible fescue grass in your pastures and hayfields. If you're "stuck" with a pasture that contains infested fescue, research has indicated that you may be able to reverse its deleterious effects by bringing your pregnant mares into stalls or drylots 60 days prior to foaling. Only fescue-free hay should be fed during these crucial 60 days, and the mares should not, under any circumstances, be

allowed to return to the pasture until after they have foaled.

7. There are many molds and fungi that can thrive in feedstuffs. Some of these contaminants are a threat to health; some are merely a detriment to the taste and/or aesthetic appearance of the food product. Unfortunately, the deadliest known contaminants can be the most difficult to see and isolate, virtually invisible to the naked eye and frustratingly elusive in the laboratory. If your feed contains corn, be aware that corn is more susceptible than most other grains to becoming contaminated with molds and fungal agents that can be very dangerous to livestock. Unfortunately, the most dangerous types of fungus on corn (*Fusarium* species, for example) are not the obvious fuzzy green stuff that is easily seen. The clinical syndrome associated with Fusarium toxicosis is the result of a toxin (poison) produced by the mold. This toxin is normally present in the mold, and as the mold goes through its life cycle and dies, its demise causes the release of the dangerous toxin. By the time the contaminated feed is consumed, the mold that produced the dangerous toxin has already disappeared.

Many of the dangerous molds and fungi can contaminate corn while it is still standing in the cornfield, some will contaminate it in the drying bins, some will contaminate it in the feed mills and some will contaminate it after it has been packaged in feed bags. The best way to be sure that the corn you're feeding is safe is to know the ultimate source and keep informed about current agricultural events. In other words, the corn being sold in feed stores in Arkansas may have been grown in Iowa or Indiana, stored in elevators in Kansas and mixed and bagged in mills in Missouri. Tracking down the ultimate source of the corn in your feed may be too difficult, in which case you may be better off using a feed that doesn't contain corn at all. Whether or not the risks are worthwhile is a personal decision that each horse owner must make individually.

Section 3.5
The Foaling Stall

The best way to avoid foal illnesses, besides adhering to good general management practices, is to provide a physically clean foaling and nursery environment that is free from current or prior exposure to other horses, particularly those which are (or have been) ill or traveling. If foaling indoors, the best stall bedding is clean, dust-free straw. **Wood shavings and/or sawdust should be strictly avoided in foaling stalls,** since the porous wood fibers are popular hiding places for some of the more virulent bacteria such as *Klebsiella* species. There is a definite correlation between increased foal illnesses and wood shavings in the foaling stall. Since newborn foals spend most of their time sleeping, nostrils at ground level, their respiratory tracts receive high exposure to the dust, spores, ammonia fumes, wood fibers and associated bacteria in moldy, dusty, dirty, urine-soaked or otherwise unsuitable bedding. Besides selecting the right kind of bedding, keeping the stall clean is also vital. Many times a stall will not seem dirty until you crouch down and take a whiff at lower levels, where the foal breathes. The ammonia fumes at the level of the foal's nostrils may be overwhelming.

The designated foaling area, whether it is a stall, paddock or pasture, should be inhabited by the mare for at least two weeks prior to foaling. This is important because every area has its own characteristic "germs" that can threaten the health of the newborn foal unless the mare is able to provide the foal with antibodies to protect him against those specific germs. The antibodies are present in the colostrum ("first milk") and will protect the foal during the first weeks of life until he is able to "build" antibodies of his own. However, even a mature horse needs at least two weeks to build antibodies against a specific germ, which is why vaccinations are not protective until two or three weeks after they are given. By the same token, if the mare is suddenly moved to the foaling stall at the moment she goes into labor, she may be completely unprepared and unable to protect her foal against the germs that unavoidably reside there. Of course any foaling area should be kept as clean as possible, preferably scrubbed and disinfected prior to putting the mare in there, and continuously stripped of manure and urine during her stay. But any germs that remain despite your good housekeeping should be protected against by colostrum from the mare, since she has had ample time to develop the necessary antibodies.

Another reason to move the mare to the foaling area two weeks before delivery is to allow her to acclimate emotionally to being separated from her herdmates. Some mares fret and pace excessively in this situation, and many people are afraid that the associated stress will cause her to foal prematurely or abort. If the foaling area is outside and is large enough, one way of dealing with this dilemma when moving the mare to the foaling area ahead of time is to allow her to bring her closest "friend" along. This is a reasonable solution, but it carries two disadvantages. First, it is essential that the foaling area be as clean as possible for the foaling, and it will be more difficult to keep it clean if there are two mares living there, not only from the standpoint of twice the manure and urine, but also because they will quickly eat up all the clean, soft grass and churn up the soil with their hooves. Secondly, it is almost without exception that the new mother will suddenly become distrustful and aggressive toward her old friend when the foal is born, and although adult horses can usually work out their differences without major injury to each other, the newborn foal is likely to get caught in the middle and can be seriously hurt or worse. If you are unlucky enough to make a quick trip to the store at the wrong time and miss the foaling, you may return to find a disaster and wish that you had never put the mares together.

Another possible solution is to design your foaling setup so that the isolated foaling mare can still see (and possibly touch noses with) her mates across a safe, sturdy barrier. If the weather forces you to foal the mare indoors, she may feel more secure if a familiar mare is in the adjacent stall. Conversely, consider that some mares have different allegiances when they have foals, and a particular individual may feel more vulnerable if there *are* other horses around. In other words, they may feel more secure if the foaling area is cozy and secluded, *away* from the other horses. In many cases, the foaling mare's rank in the herd hierarchy determines (or at least influences) her preference for privacy or for "safety in numbers." Your facility should be flexible enough to accommodate these little idiosyncrasies at a moment's notice, since in many cases the mare's whims don't become evident until the process is already under way.

Section 3.6
Supplies

Following is a list of items that should be available within easy reach of the foaling area, preferably organized in baskets or totes so that finding a specific item in a hurry is easy. Your foaling "kit" items should be stored protected from dust and dirt, for example inside plastic bags or in a closed cabinet.

> Digital readout rectal thermometer that "beeps" when ready to read
> Temperature chart, pencil
> Halter
> Lead rope
> Twitch
> Chain shank
> 2 clean buckets
> Access to warm water
> Tail wrap
> Baler's twine
> Mild liquid soap, such as Ivory
> Two 1-pound rolls of clean cotton
> Flashlight with fresh batteries
> Clean bandage scissors
> Sterile saline solution
> Wristwatch or clock
> Shoulder-length plastic gloves, sterile and individually wrapped
> Plastic garbage bags or heavy-duty empty feed sacks
> 5 tubes of sterile, nonspermicidal lubricating jelly
> Clean, soft terrycloth towels
> Clean, soft terrycloth washcloths
> Clean, lightweight cotton bedsheet

Clean cotton twine or string, a 12-inch and a 36-inch piece

Tincture of iodine (2%), 6 of the half-ounce bottles

Fleet enemas, at least 2

Sterile baby bottle with large nipple (or sheep's nipple and pop bottle)

Clean 4-cup plastic kitchen measuring container

10 pounds of fresh wheat bran

Molasses

Availability of horse trailer, preferably hooked up and ready to go

Telephone number of veterinarian, maps, gas money

"Creature comforts" (snacks, coffee, warm clothes, books, etc.)

In the freezer: frozen colostrum in case the mare has inadequate quantity or quality colostrum of her own.

Section 3.7
Basic Procedures

Prior to the foaling date, take the time and effort to learn how (and why) to do some basic procedures and to acclimate your mare to your approach and technique.

TAIL WRAPPING

There are many correct ways to wrap a tail. One method is to enclose the tail in a shoulder-length plastic glove and tie it on with a wide rubber strap at the base of the mare's tail. Another method is to use leg wraps, either the reusable or the disposable kind, and to either incorporate all the tail hairs in the wrap or to allow the long ends to hang loose. Although leaving the long ends loose is less effective in keeping the tail clean, the main purpose in wrapping the tail is to keep the *upper* hairs away from the mare's genital area so that contamination of the birth canal can be minimized. Furthermore, leaving the long ends of the tail loose allows the mare to have her "fly swatter," which is very important if the foaling is taking place during the fly season. Whatever method you choose, there are two important points to keep in mind.

First, the blood supply to the tail should not be impaired, and if your method of securing the tail wrap is applied too tightly, it can act as a tourniquet. Although it doesn't happen often, **some mares have actually lost all or part of their tails from tail wraps that were too tight and left on too long.** If your mare swishes her tail very much during the early stages of labor, she may manage to get her tail wrap off, but it is better to have the inconvenience of having to reapply the tail wrap than to have the mare's tail fall off a week later. There are tricks to getting a tail wrap to stay on without a lot of tension, and an example is offered in Figure 3.02. For best results in keeping the tail clean (which is especially important during fly season), the tail wrap should be left on until the afterbirth has passed.

Second, since the primary goal of tail wrapping is to keep hairs from touching the mare's genital area and contaminating it during labor, the wrap should incorporate the short stray hairs at the base of the tail. The tail wrap does no good in this regard if it slips down and allows the base hairs to stick out.

WASHING THE MARE'S GENITAL AREA
This should always be done gently, using a mild liquid soap (not detergent) and rinsing thoroughly. For rinsing, use a bucket of clean, warm water into which you have plunged fifteen or twenty fistfuls of cotton. Tie one end of a piece of baler's twine to the wrapped tail approximately two thirds of the way down the bony portion and tie the other end to the right side of the mare's halter, applying just enough tension to hold the tail casually to the right side. Standing just to the left, wet the vulva and about a hand's breadth of the surrounding haired skin with a wad of wet cotton, starting at the vulva and spiraling around and around, moving outward with each spiral, so that the cotton never returns to the vulva after touching the outer tissue. Discard the used cotton in a pile at your feet.

Pour about a tablespoon of Ivory liquid (soap, not detergent) into your hand and smear it gently onto the vulva, from the top to the bottom, then with the tops of your slightly bent

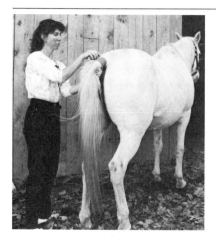
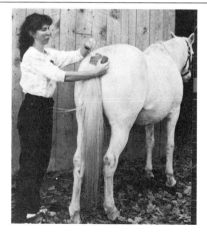

FIGURE 3.02 A,B
Using a nonadhesive leg bandage, begin the wrap at the extreme base of the tail and make one complete revolution around the tail to cover the end of the wrap. Lift up a section of tail hair and fold it up over the wrapped section.

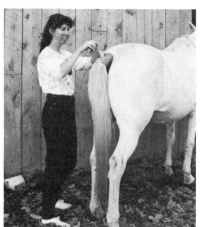
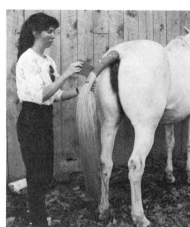

FIGURE 3.02 C,D
Continue the wrap under this raised swatch of hair, then place another revolution of the wrap over the raised swatch to secure it.

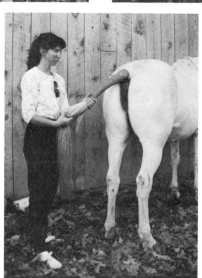

FIGURE 3.02 E
Repeat the swatch-folding process once or twice more as you move down the tail, then wrap the remaining bony part of the tail with enough tension to discourage slippage.

fingers, lather it in well, being sure to work it into the crevices on either side of the vulva. Stay away from the anus, since any contact there will only contaminate your hands and/or cotton and may cause contaminated water to drip down to the vulva from the anus. Using a fresh wad of soaked cotton each time, squeeze out the excess water so that it doesn't drip on the mare's hocks, and spiral from the vulva out, first spreading the lather to the outer area and then rinsing it off with each successive wipe. Never reuse a wad of cotton. Continue wiping until the cotton wads come away visibly clean.

WASHING THE MARE'S UDDER

As the foaling day draws near, the mare's swelling udder becomes increasingly tender, calling for especially gentle technique. However, the crevices between the two halves of the udder and between the udder and the inner surfaces of the thighs become itchy as the udder swells, since irritants such as sweat, dust and urine can no longer be "aired out" as the crevices get deeper and darker. A mild dermatitis can result, and it is not uncommon to see heavily pregnant mares straddling bushes in the pasture, rocking back and forth in an effort to scratch their itchy udders on the branches. Flies are often attracted to the damp, irritated recesses of the udders, and their bites usually create some bleeding, which invariably attracts more flies. Often the fly problem on the udder becomes so severe that the tip of the mare's tail becomes stained with blood from swishing at the flies as they continually draw blood from the besieged udder.

The blood-stained tail is often misinterpreted as a sign of a bloody vaginal discharge or bloody urine, and the veterinarian is called to examine the mare for a urogenital tract infection. If the caretaker had simply bent over and looked at the mare's udder, the diagnosis and treatment would have been obvious. A gentle washing and rinsing of the udder during these times will most likely be appreciated, and it is a good way to win the mare's trust so that you will be permitted to handle the udder when checking for milk. Furthermore, research has shown that one of the most effective ways of preventing foal diarrhea is to wash and rinse the mare's udder just prior to the foal's first milk meal. Be sure to rinse off all traces of soap.

CONFINEMENT

Although confining the mare to stanchions or stocks during gynecological procedures is almost always preferable for the operator's safety, **never put a mare in labor into a stanchion**. In some mares, the muscular and hormonal events that are taking place inside her body can hit her "like a ton of bricks," and she may collapse to the ground without notice. If she is in a stanchion when she goes down, she may break your arm or seriously injure herself, and it may be very difficult to get her back onto her feet without somebody getting hurt.

CHAPTER

4

THE FOUR PHASES OF LABOR

Section 4.1
First Phase—Pre-Stage I

Because the emerging foal in advanced labor usually presents himself to the outside world in the "diving position," it is a common misconception that he resides in the uterus in that same position: upright, nose and forelimbs aiming toward the mare's tail, crouched and ready to spring out when the time is right. In truth, during the first two-thirds of pregnancy, the fetus is in a variety of positions, "tethered" by the umbilical cord to one horn of the mare's uterus, and whether his head faces the front, back or sides of the mare is likely to be random. Recent research has shown that the normal twists in the umbilical cord are the result of the fetus rotating around the axis delineated

FIGURE 4.01
Position of the normal fetus during most of the third trimester until the beginning of labor

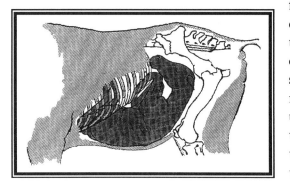

58

by the umbilical cord. The early fetus is remarkably active within the uterus, spending time in one uterine horn, then the other, rolling over, kicking, entering a uterine horn head first or tail first, spending some time apparently "sleeping" and some time moving about. As the pregnancy progresses and the fetus grows in size and weight, however, lack of space dictates that such positional changes become increasingly difficult, and an unidentified influence ensures that most fetuses spend the last one-third of pregnancy in dorsal recumbency (on their backs) with their head toward the rear of the mare, their forelimbs and nose tucked into their chest.

During the Pre-Stage I phase, which begins approximately three weeks prior to the actual birth process, the foal begins some reflex movements in preparation for the positional change he must make in order to enter the birth canal properly. He begins to extend his neck, bouncing the dorsal surface of his head on the mare's bladder, and he extends his forelimbs, essentially slapping the mare in the kidneys and colon. Each "flurry" of exercise normally lasts approximately 10 or 15 minutes. This is a time of heightened discomfort for the mare, who is already uncomfortable from the weight and increasing activity of the developing fetus.

As the Pre-Stage I exercises intensify and the fetus becomes more active, the mare is more likely to experience signs of abdominal discomfort, which can be difficult to distinguish from colic or premature labor. Increased pressure on the mare's urinary tract by the foal can make it difficult for her to urinate, and she may adopt the typical stance and strain to urinate but only manage to express a few drops of urine. As her bladder gets more distended with urine, her discomfort is magnified, and veterinary intervention becomes necessary to empty the bladder and relieve the pressure. In many cases, the fetus suddenly changes position and allows the mare to urinate on her own. In a similar scenario, the fetus may lean on a loop of the mare's bowel, temporarily pinching it closed and causing a buildup of gas.

On rare occasions, increased and intensified fetal activity during these final three weeks of pregnancy can make the mare's life so miserable that veterinary intervention is necessary to make the mare more comfortable. Sometimes, for example, the period of fetal activity lasts longer than the usual 10 or 15

During Pre-Stage I the
fetus begins stretching
and extending his neck
and forelimbs in prepa-
ration for the move-
ments he must make
during the next stage of
labor. This is essential in
order for delivery to oc-
cur without positional
error.

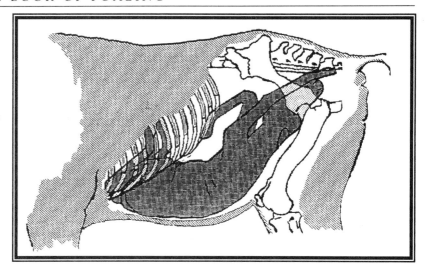

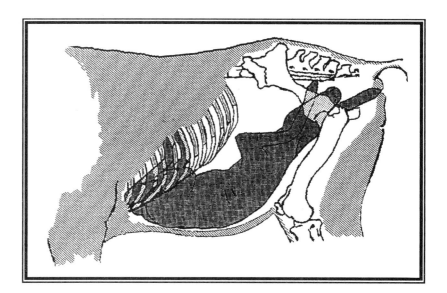

minutes, or the fetus may fall into an uncomfortable position and
struggle violently to reposition himself. In most instances, however, the increased activity of the fetus goes unnoticed by the
mare's caretakers, or is noticed only incidentally as grouchiness
or an overly active flank. **It is important to understand that the
Pre-Stage I phase is an essential component of the birthing
process, and any influence which serves to inhibit or interrupt
these reflex exercises of the fetus may contribute to a positional abnormality when real labor gets under way.**

Section 4.2

The Placenta

Before going further in the labor process, some basics about the placenta must be reviewed. The placenta is comprised functionally of two membranes—a sac within a sac.

THE ALLANTOIS-CHORION

The outer sac is called the allantois-chorion, or the allantochorionic membrane. This sac is the one that "adheres" to the mare's uterus, deriving the nutrition the fetus needs in order to survive and grow. The outer surface of the allantois-chorion is the chorionic surface, a deep-reddish-colored, roughened membrane that resembles a maroon-colored terrycloth towel. The loops of the terrycloth represent the membrane's fingerlike projections or villi. Just as the loops of the terrycloth towel increase its surface area for absorbing water, the villi of the chorionic membrane increase its surface area for absorbing oxygen and nutrient-rich blood for the fetus. These villi become embedded into the mare's uterus, each villus enveloped in its own corresponding crypt in the uterus. The attachment of villus-in-crypt is much like Velcro, a surprisingly tight attachment that can involve some bleeding when it comes apart.

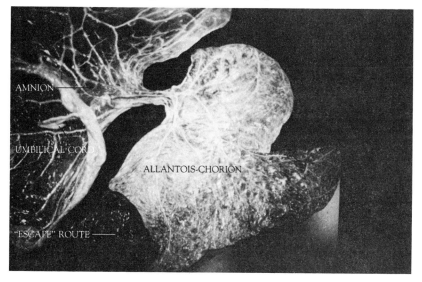

AMNION

UMBILICAL CORD

ALLANTOIS-CHORION

"ESCAPE" ROUTE

FIGURE 4.04
Entire placenta: the outer sac (allantois-chorion) and the inner sac (amnion) are indicated. Note the umbilical cord and the tear in the outer sac through which the foal "escaped."

61

FIGURE 4.05
Allantois-chorion: the outer, villus surface and the inner, smooth surface. The outer surface attaches like Velcro to the uterus in order to provide the developing fetus with blood.

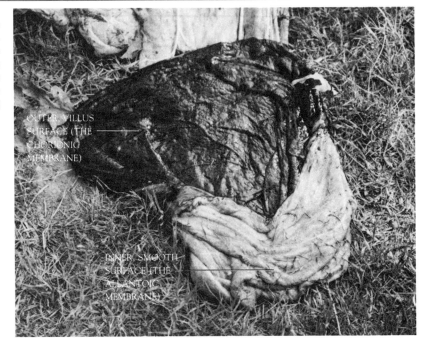

FIGURE 4.05
Allantois-chorion: the outer, villus surface and the inner, smooth surface. The outer surface attaches like Velcro to the uterus in order to provide the developing fetus with blood.

The method of attachment between the placenta and the uterus is different for different species of animals. In cows, for example, the uterus actually develops large, fleshy, oval "buttons" called caruncles, nestled into corresponding "button-holes," or cotyledons, in the placenta. The sites of attachment are the sites where the placenta gets its blood supply, much the way a tree lays down roots in the soil. In the horse, the entire placenta, rather than specific buttonlike areas of the placenta, attaches to the uterus, like Velcro, so that every square inch of placenta is attached to a corresponding square inch of uterus.

It is necessary for as much of the placenta as possible to "lay down roots" so that the developing fetus is supplied with all the nutrition it needs. If for some reason the placenta is not able to attach completely, the developing fetus will be deprived of a portion of its needed blood supply, and the result may be fetal stunting and possibly death. A uterus with a significant amount of scar tissue, for example, may not have enough healthy surface area to provide nutrition for a full-term pregnancy. Successful twin pregnancies are rare in horses for the same reason—there simply is not enough uterus to allow two entire placentas to lay down roots. There may be enough room in there for two foals,

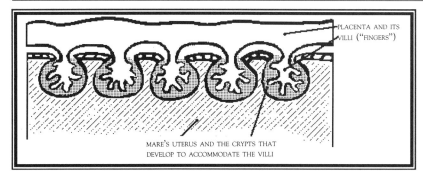

PLACENTA AND ITS VILLI ("FINGERS")

MARE'S UTERUS AND THE CRYPTS THAT DEVELOP TO ACCOMMODATE THE VILLI

FIGURE 4.06
Schematic diagram of placental "fingers" and the manner in which they embed into the uterus to attach, Velcro-style.

but each placenta is much larger than the fetus it houses, and every square inch of that placenta must be allowed to attach, like Velcro, to uterine surface. If a twin pregnancy is allowed to become established, a competition for uterine surface area ensues, and if a live birth is produced, usually at least one of the foals will be stunted or dead due to inadequate nutrition during development.

THE AMNION

The inner sac of the equine placenta is called the amnion. This is a much thinner, more delicate, milky-white-colored membrane that appears at the lips of the mare's vulva during the birthing process. When the outer sac, the allantois-chorion, ruptures and releases the allantoic fluid ("breaking the water"), the amnion advances to the vulva. The fetus is housed within the amnion, and the translucency of the milky-white amnion makes it possible to see the foal's feet through the membrane.

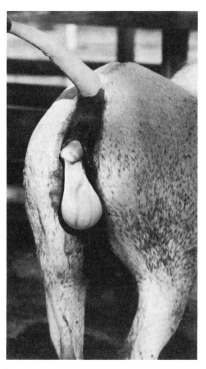

FIGURE 4.07
The amnion is the thin, milky-white inner sac that advances to the vulva within five minutes after the outer sac (the allantois-chorion) ruptures and releases the allantoic fluid ("breaking water"). Notice that the foal's hoof is visible through the translucent amnion in this mare.

63

FIGURE 4.08
The amnion encases the foal like a flimsy nightgown.

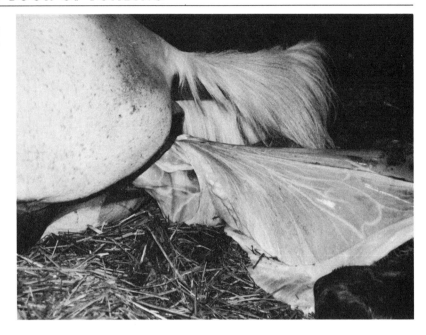

FIGURE 4.09
This mare has completed delivery and her newborn foal is lying in the lower right corner of the photo. Notice that the allantois-chorion (the "purple part") is visible protruding from the vulva, just to the left of the amnion.

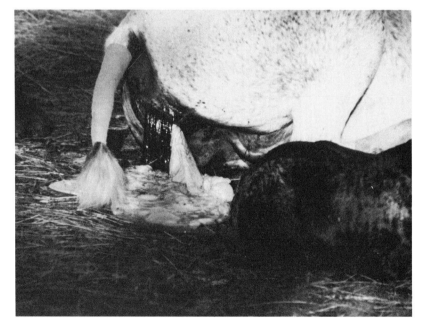

Section 4.3
Second Phase—Stage 1

Stage I of labor is that magical time of anticipation and excitement when the mare may exhibit any or all of a list of symptoms including restlessness, anxiety, loss of appetite, tail swishing, kicking at her belly, sweating in the flanks and armpits, looking at or biting at her flanks, cramping, frequently passing small amounts of loose manure, repeatedly lying down and getting up, pressing her tail against a fence or other solid object and separating herself from pasturemates.

This is another area where a common misconception prevails—that the mare's discomfort during Stage I is the result of uterine contractions. This misconception has been upheld by the observation that a mare may "grunt" every 5 seconds when she lies down during the last few weeks of pregnancy, fooling the attendant into thinking that she has gone into labor and is having contractions every 5 seconds. This is an extrapolation from human obstetrics that does not apply to the equine. The grunting is the result of the increased size and weight of the mare's abdomen pressing against her diaphragm when she lies down, making it difficult for her to breathe. Since the normal respiratory rate of a horse at rest is approximately 12 breaths per minute, a rhythmic grunting once every 5 seconds is logically her attempt to breathe, not uterine contractions.

In fact, uterine contractions in the mare are the result of the presence of the hormone oxytocin, and research has shown that there is relatively little oxytocin in the mare's bloodstream during Stage I of labor. The signs exhibited by the mare during Stage I are the result of the hormone prostaglandin, which is released in connection with the opening of the cervix, that anterior barrier to the birth canal. Any woman who has ever had an intrauterine device (IUD) installed for birth control may recall the pain involved when her gynecologist mechanically dilated (stretched) the cervix to admit the IUD. The discomfort is the result of prostaglandin released from the mechanically disturbed cervix. Another illustration of the effects of prostaglandin is the classical response of mares to an injection of the estrus-synchronizing drug prostaglandin F2 alpha (brand names

Prostin or Lutalyse, manufactured by Upjohn). Although there are synthetic drugs now available that serve a similar purpose but which have fewer uncomfortable side effects, veterinarians will choose the natural products for selected cases, and the temporary side effects are predictable: restlessness, anxiety, passing small amounts of increasingly wet manure, tail swishing, kicking at the belly, sweating, looking at the flanks, cramping, lying down, getting up, lying down, getting up—all the classic symptoms of so-called "labor" in a mare that isn't even pregnant. Prostaglandin causes these symptoms, not oxytocin. **The mare in Stage I of labor is not having labor contractions**, and this is one of the most important points to remember when learning how to attend foalings effectively.

During Stage I of labor, the mare's discomfort stems from the gradual opening of the cervix. While the cervix is opening, some very important progress is being made inside the uterus where the placenta and fetus reside. The pregnancy, which consists of an 80- to 120-pound foal, several heavy gallons of fluid and two heavy sacks, is much like a very full, very heavy water balloon. If you hold a water balloon in your hands and attempt to throw it, you may find that the weight of the water will break the balloon in your arms before your throw is complete. If, however, you are able to support the water balloon on all surfaces so that no single area of the balloon becomes overly stretched while you execute your throw, the balloon is less likely to tear prematurely. Imagine that you've placed the water balloon into a pillowcase. The fabric of the pillowcase helps to support the fragile walls of the balloon, preventing the water inside from stretching the balloon's walls beyond their limit, and you should be able to swing it about and carry it much more casually, knowing that it is much less likely to break accidentally. By the same token, the uterus supports the somewhat unstable walls of the placenta so that the weight of the foal and all that fluid is much less likely to rupture the placenta prematurely.

During Stage I of labor, however, the cervix is opening, and suddenly the placenta is no longer supported on all surfaces—suddenly there is an unsupported spot. As the cervix continues to open wider, the unsupported area grows larger, and all the weight of the pregnancy begins to be transmitted to that spot, pouching through the ever-widening opening, stretching thinner and thinner as the weight of the fluid begins to shift. Cleverly enough, if everything is in the proper alignment, the portion of the placenta that abuts against the opening cervix and bulges through it happens to be a thinner, weaker spot in the placenta. This portion of the placenta is called the "cervical star," because it abuts against the cervix, and because it looks like a star. When the cervix has opened widely enough to expose the margins of the cervical star, the bulging placenta should rupture at that weak spot, and the gallons of liquid inside will come gushing or trickling out, depending on the mare's position and the size of the rupture. This is called "breaking the water," and it marks the end of Stage I and the beginning of Stage II of labor.

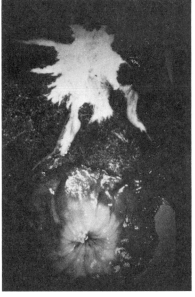

FIGURE 4.10
Cervix (below) removed and placed next to the cervical star portion of a placenta

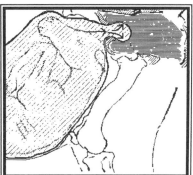

FIGURE 4.11
Diagram of the allantois-chorion protruding through the opening cervix

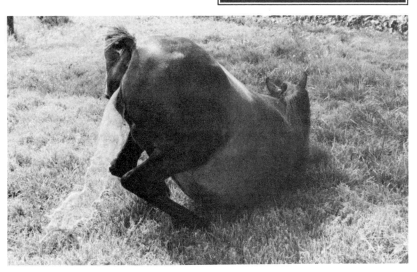

FIGURE 4.12
When the water breaks, the allantoic fluid comes out forcibly or in a trickle, depending on the position of the mare and the amount of pressure on the uterus at the time the cervical star ruptures.

67

Occasionally there may be a problem with the rupturing of the cervical star. Perhaps the cervical star does not align perfectly with the cervix, causing the weak spot in the placenta to lie off center with the opening cervix. Or perhaps the placenta is thickened as a result of a disease process or a nutritional imbalance, and the thickened placenta is too tough to rupture when it protrudes through the opening cervix. Whatever the cause, if the mare should fail to "break the water" before going into serious labor contractions, a dangerous situation will result, and you should be ready to recognize this situation and correct it immediately—early detection and early correction.

FIGURE 4.13
As the opening in the cervix widens, the unsupported fluid-filled allantois-chorion begins to protrude into the vagina and finally ruptures.

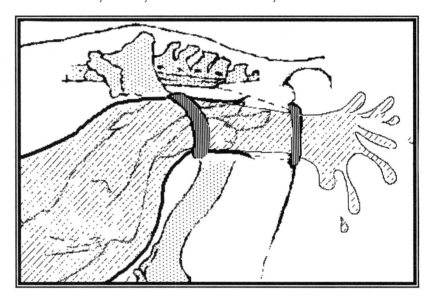

In the normal situation, when the outer placental sac ruptures at the cervical star, the inner sack (amnion) should then be allowed to advance and should appear at the vulvar lips of the mare within 5 minutes. Remember that the allantois-chorion (the outer sac) is a dark red, roughened, terrycloth-like membrane, and the amnion is thinner, more delicate and translucent milky-white in color.

It is important to note that the opening of the cervix is not an isolated event—it would not occur if not for the pressure exerted on it by the stretching foal. Rather, the cervix softens and becomes pliable, thereby allowing the foal to push through and stretch it open. On rare occasions the stretching foal is out of alignment, and instead of pressing through the cervix, the foal's forelimbs press against the wall of the vagina adjacent to the cervix, much the same way a performer would struggle to walk off stage when he can't find the opening in the stage drapery. A mare in this situation will display an abnormally prolonged Stage I and may be headed for trouble if a knowledgeable attendant isn't around. To correct the problem, the veterinarian simply reaches into the vagina, through the flabby (but undistended) cervix and grasps the foal's front hooves, redirecting them through the cervix as the hand is withdrawn.

If for some reason the allantois-chorion does not rupture as it should, the mare will do one of two things: she will either stop

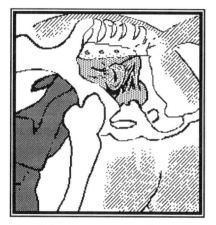 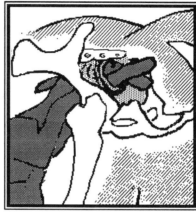

FIGURE 4.14 A,B
The foal's limbs can be out of alignment with the cervix, pressing on the wall of the vagina next to the cervix. Manually redirecting them through the cervix resolves the problem.

the labor process and start again later, or she will begin the uterine contractions of serious labor and try to push the pregnancy out in its entirety—the foal, the amnion, the amniotic fluid, the allantoic fluid and the allantois-chorion—she will try to force the entire, intact water balloon and its gallons of fluid out through the rigid walls of the birth canal. This is called a "dry birth."

DRY BIRTH

A dry birth is dangerous to the foal for two reasons, besides the obvious disadvantage of the lack of lubrication. First, as a result of that lack of lubrication in concert with the increase in size of the overall "package" due to the fact that the whole placental unit is trying to come out at the same time as the foal, the foal is being subjected to a tremendous increase in pressure and stress, leaving it more susceptible to physical and neurological damage.

Second, think about the source of the foal's oxygen—the fetus receives its oxygen not from *breathing*, but rather from the *blood of his dam*. When the fetus emerges from the mare, his former oxygen source is cut off, and he must learn to breathe on his own in order to oxygenate his own blood.

But before he emerges, while he's still inside the mare, where does the blood in his umbilical artery come from? It comes from the little "roots" of the placenta that are embedded into the uterus, drawing blood from the blood supply of the mare's uterus. If the allantois-chorion fails to rupture and the mare's uterus begins to contract, eventually she will manage to push the pregnancy far enough out so that you can see the chorionic surface of the placenta at the lips of the vulva. This means that it has begun to detach from its Velcro-like attachment in the uterus (premature separation), so that at least a portion of the placenta is now no longer drawing blood from the uterus because it is no longer attached. So now the baby is no longer receiving his full ration of blood and oxygen. As the mare continues to push, more and more of the placenta will come apart from the uterus, and the baby will receive less and less oxygen. If this is allowed to continue for too long, the foal will suffocate, since it is caught in limbo between umbilical oxygenation and air breath-

FIGURE 4.15
The allantois-chorion has failed to rupture, and the force of the uterine contractions has pushed the pregnancy and both intact sacs to the vulva. Note that instead of the thin, milky amnion, the membrane that appears is the thick, roughened, dark red allantois-chorion.

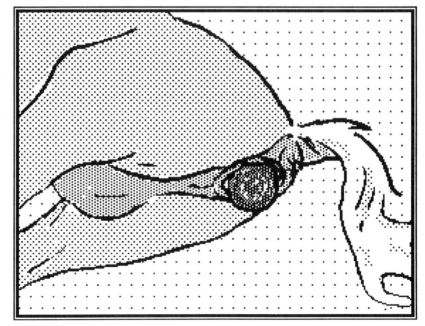

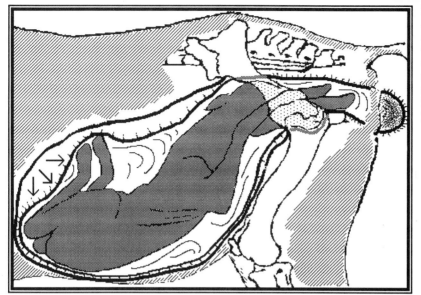

FIGURE 4.16
As the allantois-chorion detaches from the uterus, the foal is gradually deprived of oxygen and will suffocate if something isn't done immediately to stop the premature separation.

ing. And all of this is happening during a time when the foal can least afford to be deprived of oxygen, since he's in the middle of a terribly stressful situation: birth.

If the situation is corrected in time to save the foal's life but not soon enough to prevent him from being deprived of oxygen for a significant period of time, he may survive, but he will exhibit a degree of brain damage as a result of the ordeal. His symptoms may range from being "just a little slow" (known as a "dummy foal") to blindness, convulsions and coma. Armed with just a little knowledge, you can catch this problem early and correct it before any damage is done. Obviously there is not time to wait for help to arrive.

So what do you do?

Do you push the pregnancy back in so that it doesn't come away from the uterus any farther? Absolutely not. The power of the uterine contractions would be impossible to overcome, and your efforts would only result in the mare pushing even harder.

Do you grab the exposed membranes and pull the pregnancy out so that the foal can "air breathe?" This would also be virtually impossible, and it would result in significant damage to the mare's birth canal. Furthermore, by the time you succeeded in extracting the foal it would probably be dead. Remember, you'd not only be pulling the weight of the foal but also up to 75

71

pounds of liquid and placental membranes through a canal that is barely large enough to admit the foal alone.

The solution to the problem is very simple. First, be there when the mare foals. Watch for the water breaking. Whenever she lies down, walk around to a position where you can see her vulva. If you see the allantois-chorion at the vulva (remember what it looks like!), use whatever is handy—a knife, a pair of scissors, your fingers, whatever—and break it open. The allantoic fluid ("water") will come out through the tear you've created, and the birthing will proceed. It's that simple. By simply being there and knowing what to watch for, you can save the day with this simple procedure.

FIGURE 4.17
When necessary, manually rupturing the abnormally thick allantois-chorion will permit the allantoic fluid to escape ("break water") and will arrest premature separation of the placenta from the uterus.

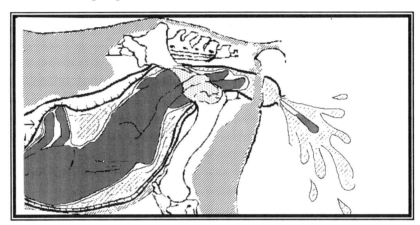

OPENING THE CASLICK'S
Although it's definitely late to be considering this, many people get preoccupied with the responsibilities of foaling and forget to have their mares' Caslick's closures opened. Under certain circumstances, the upper two-thirds of the mare's vulva is sutured (stitched) closed, leaving just enough of the lower portion open to permit urination. There can be merits to this procedure, but it is a procedure that is surely done more often than is warranted by the mare's anatomy. The vulva is supposed to form a seal or barrier against contamination of the vagina by the outside world. Sometimes it is an ineffective barrier, either because of the mare's natural anatomy or because of scar tissue from injury and/or numerous previous Caslick's operations. Routinely suturing all mares, even the two-year-olds, in the belief that this will

ensure their reproductive futures simply doesn't make any sense. Racehorses, on the other hand, may "suck wind" into their vaginas while running, especially when muscle fatigue sets in. When sutured, these mares seem to run better, and they also have fewer problems with infection when they enter their breeding years. If the mare in your care has been sutured, the vulva will have to be cut open prior to foaling. Otherwise, the emerging foal will cause the mare's vulva to rip in a random fashion, often causing considerable damage to the structure of the vulva.

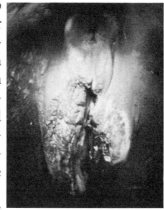

FIGURE 4.18
If a Caslick's closure is not opened prior to foaling, the vulva, which will tear, may not tear on the sutureline. This vulva was severely damaged because the mare foaled before the Caslick's closure was opened.
(Photo courtesy of Dr. W.T.K. Bosu, University of Wisconsin School of Veterinary Medicine, Madison, Wisconsin)

Although a few nonveterinarians seem to enjoy doing this procedure themselves, without benefit of local anesthesia or clean surgical instruments, the safest and most humane way to open a Caslick's closure is to have a veterinarian numb the area with injections of a local anesthetic agent and cut the line open with surgical scissors or a scalpel. And since mares have been known to foal earlier than expected, do not postpone opening a Caslick's closure until very close to the anticipated foaling date. **Have all Caslick's closures opened on the 300th day of the pregnancy.** Be prepared for anything, however, because if you are attending a mare already in the first stages of labor and you suddenly discover that she has a closed Caslick's sutureline, you will have to take the responsibility to open her up yourself. Obviously this is a situation best avoided by having the presence of mind to attend to it beforehand.

The best time to perform an emergency opening of a Caslick's sutureline is during the actual delivery of the foal. At this time, the sensitivity of the vulvar tissue to painful stimuli is somewhat dulled, and the mare, preoccupied with the pain of labor, is unlikely to resent having the sutureline cut. Insert two fingers behind the sutureline and pull it slightly toward you so that the underlying structures (and the foal) are not poked or cut by the scissors. Before you begin cutting, examine the vulva closely and determine how far toward the anus your cut should extend. Use clean, sharp bandage scissors, and try to stay precisely on the midline, since this will minimize bleeding and pain.

73

Remember to watch your mares closely throughout the *early* stages of the third trimester of pregnancy too, just in case a mare is having a problem with her pregnancy and preparing to abort. If this is going to happen, there's probably a good reason for it, and most attempts to halt the abortion are likely to be unsuccessful. More important, however, is the welfare of the mare if she was previously Caslick's sutured—her vulva is almost certain to be torn if a late abortion occurs when the fetus is close to full size. Even though the odds of your mare aborting are pretty slim, it is your responsibility to keep the possibility in mind, especially if your mare is sutured. Remember that her body may tell you if she's getting ready to abort—even if the foal is seriously premature—and, if nothing more, you can take steps to protect her from damage or injury as a result of the situation. What do you do? You stay with her, ready to open the sutureline if she begins to abort. Better yet, you call your veterinarian to examine the mare to see if there's anything that can be done to prevent the abortion, and, just in case, you have the Caslick's sutureline opened.

Section 4.4
Third Phase—Stage II, the Beginning

The beginning of Stage II is marked by the rupturing of the allantois-chorion ("breaking of the water"), whether the allantois-chorion ruptures spontaneously or whether you do it manually. It is important to remember that **true labor contractions have not yet begun**, and any positional abnormalities of the foal must be corrected *now*, before the mare begins to push. Although I am a firm advocate of being conservative in our intrusions into the mare's natural processes, you must assume some of the responsibility for the risks to which you have exposed your mare by breeding her, and part of assuming that risk involves manually invading the birth canal. The best way to prevent harm to the mare during foaling, besides consistently providing optimal health and nutritional care and sensible exercise, is to be with her during the foaling process and to check the foal's position before true labor begins. This is a relatively invasive procedure that can be an intimidating experience for the novice, but with proper organization and preparation it can be done quickly and safely.

As a rule, there is a lag period of approximately 5 minutes between breaking water and full labor, and any manipulations in the vagina may well stimulate the mare to begin labor earlier. This gives the foaling attendant a small but usually adequate period of time to check the position of the foal and make any necessary

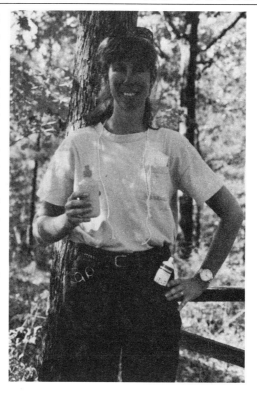

FIGURE 4.19
The essential items for the immediate foaling period should be on your person, not fifteen feet away in a basket. Carry at least two individually wrapped sterile shoulder-length disposable gloves, sterile lubricating jelly, a 12-inch piece and a 36-inch piece of clean cotton string, clean bandage scissors and your surgical iodine solution for treating the fresh umbilical stump.

corrections. By the time this moment arrives, you should be completely prepared by having all the items you may need easily within your reach. The most important things to have in your pockets are your individually wrapped sterile gloves, sterile lubricating jelly (be sure to open the sealed nozzle ahead of time), a 12-inch piece of clean cotton string, a 36-inch piece of clean cotton string, clean bandage scissors and your iodine solution for treating the fresh umbilical stump.

As soon as the water breaks, prepare to check for foal position. If the mare is lying down, she may permit you to do the entire procedure without getting up. But be ready to move out of the way in a hurry if she suddenly gets a cramp and decides to roll over onto her back—you may get hit in the face by a hoof or a hock if you're slow to move. It is generally safer if the mare is standing, although there is always the danger of being kicked if the mare is irritable or if your technique is less than gentle. Never assume that a mare will not kick because she's "sweet" or because she knows you—these are extenuating circumstances, to say the least, and a mare may not behave in the manner to which you've become accustomed. As a rule, however, even mares that are ordinarily touchy about their back ends are exceptionally tolerant of vaginal invasion when they are in the process of giving birth.

With a trusted, attentive partner at the mare's head, resecure the mare's tail wrap if it has come loose or if stray hairs have managed to work their way out. If necessary, tie a light rope or heavy string (such as baler's twine) to the knot at the end of the wrapped tail and tie the other end to the mare's halter, putting just enough tension on it to hold the tail gently off to one side. Be sure to tie onto the hair of the tail, not the living bony or fleshy portion.

Using a bucket of clean warm water and several wads of clean cotton, gently but quickly wash the mare's vulva. Place a teaspoon or so of Ivory liquid soap (not detergent) in your hand and briskly massage it onto the mare's wetted vulva until it is well lathered. Then, using a fresh wad of soaked cotton each time, rinse and rinse until the vulva is squeaky clean. Check each wad of cotton after you've wiped the mare to see if it is soiled. You are not finished until the cotton wads are clean after

FIGURE 4.20 A,B
Example of accepted procedure for washing the mare's perineal area: with a trusted attendant at the mare's head, the tail is wrapped and tied over to one side. Then the vulva is gently but thoroughly washed and rinsed.

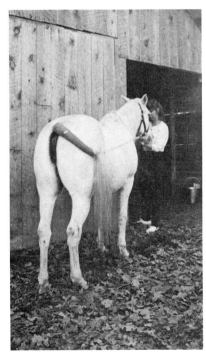
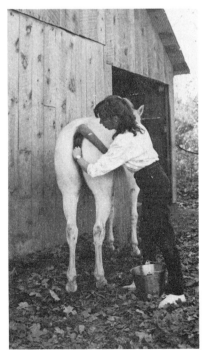

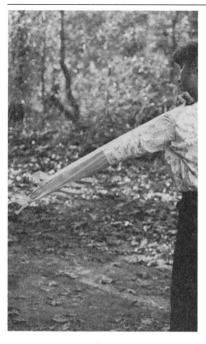

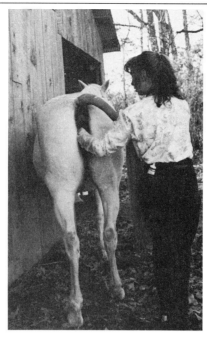

FIGURE 4.21 A,B
Being careful not to allow the sterile glove to touch any nonsterile surface, remove it from its wrapping, put it on and generously apply sterile lubricant.

Always standing off to one side, gently insert your flat hand through the vulva, relax your fingers and locate the foal's muzzle and both front hooves.

wiping the mare. However, do not get "wrapped up" in this procedure and waste time—it is very important to get the mare clean, but the whole process of washing should take no more than a minute.

Being careful not to contaminate your sterile glove by allowing it to drift or blow against a nonsterile surface, pull it on and generously lubricate your gloved hand, wrist and forearm on both sides with the sterile lube. Don't spread it around with your other hand, and don't forget to remove your wristwatch and any jewelry that may protrude and cause abrasions. With your fingers and thumb pressed together and your hand in a flattened position, gently slide your hand into the vulva. Allow your hand to relax and become accustomed to its surroundings. In many cases, the foal's fore-

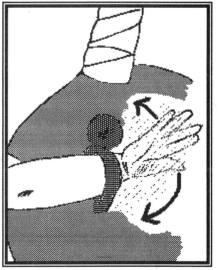

FIGURE 4.22
Gently sweep your flattened but relaxed hand to one side along the floor, up the wall, halfway across the ceiling and then back down to the floor to climb the opposite wall.

limbs are already advanced to the vulva, but sometimes you must gently press your relaxed hand farther into the vagina before locating the foal's hooves. Keeping in mind that one hoof should be about three to six inches behind the other, and that the foal's nose should be another two inches behind that, gently locate and identify the parts. If something is missing, search the vagina again—even though it's relatively small and crowded in there, it's amazing how easily a hoof or a muzzle can hide. The best way to search without wasting time is to sweep your flattened hand to one side along the floor, up the wall, halfway across the ceiling and then back down to the floor to climb the opposite wall in the same manner.

If everything is completely normal, you will find two front hooves and one muzzle—no more, no less. When satisfied that the right parts are present and accounted for, withdraw your hand, remove your glove, untie the mare's tail (but leave it wrapped), release the mare and back off.

If there's a positional abnormality, your job is usually only slightly more involved. Think about what the normal situation would be like, then decide how this situation differs from the normal. Realize that any abnormality can lead to dystocia (difficult birth). Your veterinarian should be on the way, but this can't wait, so you will have to get started. The first thing to do is to identify the problem.

Section 4.5
Stage II, Dystocia

1. There are two hooves, but you can't find the muzzle
It's probably there, but you have to go in a little farther to find it. If the foal is upside down, which is common and usually nothing to worry about (discussed later in this section), the muzzle will be under the limbs instead of above them.

Sometimes, however, the neck is either bent way back or bent forward with the head tucked into the foal's chest, and you will have to locate the head and bring it into the birth canal in order for the foal to be delivered without harm. Don't panic. Run your relaxed hand up the inner surface of one of the legs, which will lead you to the anterior portion of the foal's chest. Then, maintaining constant contact with the foal so your hand doesn't get "lost," run your hand up to the front surface of the neck. Follow the neck to the head—the head is

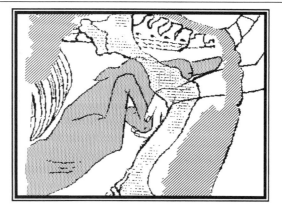

FIGURE 4.23
Sometimes the neck is bent and the head is trapped in the mare's abdomen, making it necessary to go in after it. The head is identified by the lower jaw bones, the muzzle and teeth, or the ears.

easily identified by the two big jaw bones (mandibles), or by the ears, depending on where your hand is. Follow the length of the head to the muzzle, which you can identify by slipping your finger or thumb into the foal's mouth. With your hand in the foal's mouth, grasp the chin or the upper part of the jaw, whichever is easier to reach, and use it as your handle to bring the foal's head into the birth canal.

Sometimes the reason you can't find the head is because the foal is backwards. You will discover this when you find that the soles of the feet are facing up instead of down (which is not *always* an indicator of trouble) *and* when you run your hand midway up the leg and find a rear-leg hock joint instead of a foreleg carpus (the front "knee"), and when instead of finding the chest and neck between the legs, you find a tail. You can't turn the foal around to deliver nose first; you'll have to resign yourself to a butt-first delivery and make the best of it. If the tail

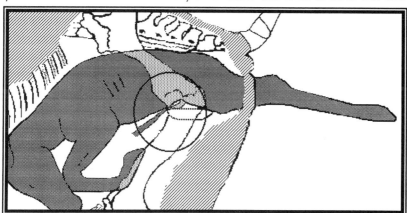

FIGURE 4.24
If the foal is backwards, he will be at increased risk of suffocation during delivery because of the increased pressure on the umbilical cord as it becomes pinched on the mare's pelvic rim.

79

is on the bottom instead of on the top, the foal is not only backwards, it's also upside down. This is not a situation for the weak at heart, so it's better to get the mare up and try to walk her, preferably downhill, to try and postpone delivery until the veterinarian arrives. If she won't be put off, however, and insists on going into delivery before professional help is available, you will have to do the best you can to help her. **This is one of those rare instances where the foal should be pulled out as quickly as possible,** because once the foal starts coming out, the weight of its body will pinch the umbilical cord against the brim of the mare's pelvis, essentially suffocating the foal. With your clean, gloved hand, slather the pelvic brim of the mare and as much as possible of the foal (inside the mare) with sterile lube. You will need to use several tubes of lube, and be quick about it.

When the mare starts to push, help her by pulling on the legs. If the foal is upside down, apply torsion (rotational force)

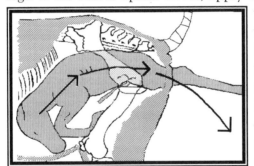

FIGURE 4.25
The arc-like direction of the foal's delivery must be kept in mind, especially when pulling the backwards foal. Otherwise severe damage can be done to both the mare and the foal.

to the foal as well as traction (pulling) by crossing the legs and trying to rotate the foal into the proper presentation (back up, stomach down, parallel to the mare). When the foal is right side up, direct your pull out and slightly down, realizing that the foal must follow an arc-like path in order to safely navigate the pelvic canal. Assume that the foal will be oxygen-deprived when it emerges, and be prepared to administer oxygen or mouth-to-nose resuscitation (see Section 5.4 on caring for the at-risk foal).

Realize also that the backwards delivery of a foal puts the mare at considerable risk of uterine tearing or rupture. She will need immediate veterinary attention to determine if this has happened and to prevent the serious and often fatal complications that arise.

2. You find the muzzle, but no hooves

This is not as bad as it sounds, because at least you know the foal is not backwards. With your relaxed hand, identify the foal's chin, and run your hand along the lower jaw to the neck, down

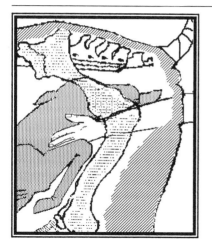 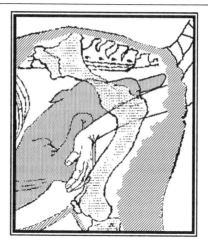

FIGURE 4.26 A,B
By running the hand along the underside of the foal's neck, the shoulder and then the elbow of the retained limb can be located.

the neck to the chest, then over to one side, where you'll find the elbow. Cup your hand under the elbow, then run it along the underside of the forearm until you get to the fetlock joint. Grasp the fetlock joint, flexing it so the hoof is flexed back against the forearm, and bring the flexed fetlock and hoof up and toward you, over the pelvic brim and into the pelvic canal alongside the head. Repeat with the other side. Some operators find it easier to bring the leg into the pelvic canal by grasping the toe of the hoof instead of the fetlock, which is fine, but sometimes the toe is just a little too far away, and the fetlock is within reach.

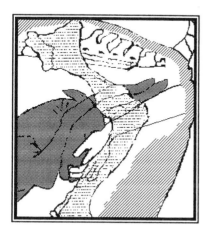 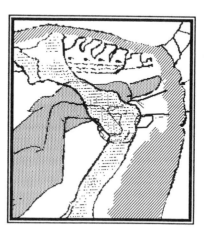

FIGURE 4.27 A,B
By following the limb down from the elbow, the "knee" (carpus) can be bent and the fetlock and hoof reached, cupped in the hand to protect the mare and brought up and into the birth canal.

The most important things to remember are to be careful to protect the mare's uterus from puncture or rupture by sharp points, such as little hooves or your fingers, and to contaminate the mare's vaginal and uterine cavities as little as possible.

81

3. You find the muzzle and only one hoof

Using the same technique as in #2 above, figure out which leg is missing and retrieve it.

4. You find the muzzle and three hooves

The trick here is to figure out which leg(s) is a rear leg and which ones are forelimbs. Usually in a case like this, the foal is *almost* in the proper position but one of the rear legs has gotten caught over the pelvic brim and is now crowding the pelvic canal. This is commonly referred to as "dog-sitting." You can either try to identify the rear leg by running your hand up each leg looking for a hock joint, or try to identify the forelegs by running your hand up the legs to the chest that "connects" them. Once you've identified the "extra" leg, cup your hand over the sharp tip of the hoof and escort the leg back over the pelvic brim into the abdomen.

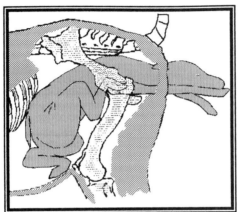

FIGURE 4.28
"Dog-sitting" foal. One or both hind limbs is caught on the mare's pelvic rim. Once the "extra" limb has been identified, it must be escorted over the pelvic rim and released back into the abdomen.

Hopefully you will never be in a situation where the third leg belongs to a twin foal. At this stage in the art of veterinary medicine, the diagnosis of twin pregnancies is readily and easily done by ultrasound examination, and steps can be taken to be sure one of the twins is eliminated early in the game. There is really no good excuse today for exposing a mare to the often fatal hazard of carrying twin fetuses all the way to term, but if you should inherit such a problem by acquiring a pregnant mare that was not properly monitored by ultrasound during the early stages of her pregnancy, you may be presented with a hopeless tangle of legs during the delivery. Remarkably, many of the rare twin deliveries that do occur tend to proceed without getting tangled up. But if there is a tangle, you and your veterinarian will have a tense and challenging situation that will rival even the most difficult jigsaw puzzles. The twin delivery is mentioned here only so that you will not fail to *consider* it as a possibility if you identify a positional abnormality during delivery.

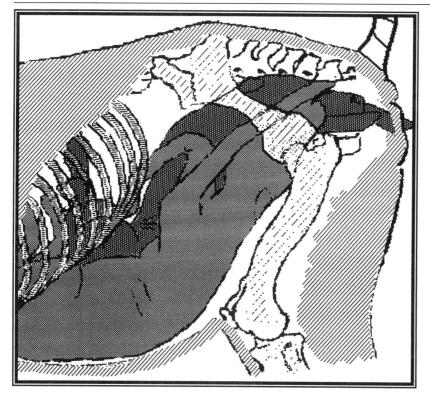

FIGURE 4.29
Term twin pregnancy, where the attendant must discern which legs belong to which foal before delivery can proceed.

5. You find the muzzle, but instead of two hooves, there are "knees"

In this situation, the forelimbs (one or both) accidentally got bent while entering the pelvic canal, so instead of presenting toe first, the involved leg presents "knee" (carpus) first. This is the situation that the foal's exercises during Pre-Stage I were designed to prevent. The problem with this position is that the hoof, which is now back in the mare's abdomen against the foal's chest area, makes that portion of the foal too big to fit easily through the pelvic canal, because it will

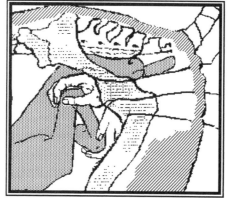

FIGURE 4.30
When one or both "knees" (carpi) are bent, the knee must be pushed in and up to bring the retained hoof up into the birth canal. If necessary, and if the mare is large enough, a second hand can be inserted into the vagina to retrieve the hoof once it has reached the pelvic rim.

come through at the same time as the foal's chest, elbows and shoulders. It would be a mistake to try to straighten the leg by

83

reaching all the way into the mare's uterus to find the foal's hoof and trying to bring it toward you. There simply is not enough room in the pelvic canal for you to manipulate the foal's leg this way while your arm is alongside the foal's torso. The easiest way to straighten the leg is to grasp the "knee" and push it *in and up* toward the ceiling of the mare's pelvis. Unless the foal's legs are very long, this should bring the hoof into the pelvic canal so that you can grasp it with your other hand, cupping the tip of the hoof in your hand to protect the mare, and bring it toward you into position.

6. You find nothing—no muzzle, no hooves, nothing!
Check again—are you sure? This could be one of those very dangerous situations called transverse presentation, meaning that the foal is sideways and can't fit into the pelvic canal at all. The only way to resolve this situation safely is by cesarean section.

Another possibility is that the foal is deformed somehow, such as having an extremely enlarged head or a very crooked neck and/or legs. In most cases like this, the foal can only be delivered by cesarean, and the surgery is necessary to save the mare. Extreme cases are resolved by fetotomy, whereby the foal is cut up and delivered through the pelvic canal in pieces, but this is extremely dangerous and hazardous to the mare's life and future as a broodmare, and obviously both procedures are to be handled only by qualified veterinary surgeons. The only way to prepare for such situations is to have your horse trailer hooked up and ready to roll, your route planned and the surgeon's telephone number posted by the phone. Don't make any decisions one way or the other until your regular veterinarian has had a chance to make a careful diagnosis.

A less dangerous possibility is that the foal is slightly out of alignment and instead of pressing against the cervix, forcing it open and gaining entrance into the birth canal, the foal is pressing into one of the lateral edges of the vaginal wall adjacent to the cervix. An illustrative analogy is the child trying to get his arms into the sleeves of a cardigan sweater—he thrusts his hand in what he perceives to be the location of the sleeve entrance, but he's off the mark, and his hand merely stretches the fabric adjacent to the armhole. The child's predicament is resolved when his mother inserts her hand up the sleeve from the cuff to the armhole, grasps his searching hand and leads it back out through the sleeve. In the case of the foal, the attendant must insert a hand into the vagina and through the cervix and identify the parts of the foal that lie beyond. When the muzzle and forelimbs are found, slightly off axis to one side or the other, they should be directed through the cervix into the birth canal and the delivery should proceed normally.

Finally, and most dangerously for mare and foal, if no hooves or muzzle are located in the birth canal, it is possible that the mare's uterus has undergone twisting (torsion). This twists the exit closed, the same way that twisting a large sack full of leaves closes the top of the sack and keeps the leaves from coming out. Most cases of uterine torsion require surgery to be re-

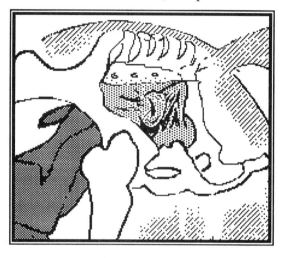

FIGURE 4.31
The foal's muzzle and forelimbs may be slightly out of alignment with the mare's cervix, pressing in vain against the soft forward wall of the birth canal formed by the anterior wall of the vagina.

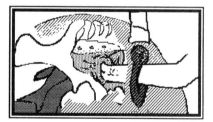 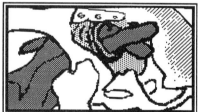

FIGURE 4.32 A,B
The problem is easily re-solved by manually guiding the foal's muzzle and forelimbs through the cervix into the birth canal.

solved, and the risk to the mare in these surgeries is significant because of the effects of the torsion on her circulatory system. The longer the delay between the occurrence of the torsion and the surgery, the more difficult the surgery will be on the mare. Saving the foal in these cases is very difficult and is usually not possible, since the blood supply to the uterus is impaired by the torsion.

Some torsions have successfully been resolved by rolling the mare in the direction of the torsion. This is possible only if the mare has not yet suffered any serious damage as a result of the torsion (such as ruptured vaginal or uterine tissue) and if the direction of the twist can be determined. If the uterus has twisted in a clockwise direction, for example, the goal is to lay the anesthetized mare on her right side and roll her legs up and over in a clockwise direction while attempting to hold the heavy uterus back with a large weighted plank. General anesthesia is mandatory, as is absolute certainty that the direction of the torsion is known; otherwise this procedure may only worsen the situation.

FIGURE 4.33
If the uterus is twisted in a clockwise direction, the anesthetized mare is positioned on her right side with a weighted plank resting on her abdomen to hold the foal in place. The goal is to rotate the mare around the uterus to reestablish normal position.

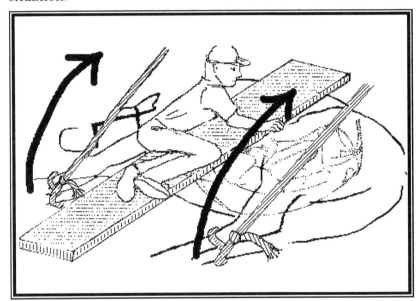

7. The foal is not responding properly

On rare occasions, the foal is not receiving the proper "signals," either because there is something wrong with his central nervous system, or because the signals themselves are being garbled somehow. In some cases, for example, the foal may be in exactly the right position, but when the mare's uterus begins to tense and push against him, he reacts inappropriately by arching his neck and tucking his nose into his chest. When the contractions cease, the foal relaxes and appears to be in the proper position, but as soon as the contractions resume, the foal arches up again and makes it impossible for his head to enter the birth canal. In cases like this, oftentimes there are additional indications that the foal is abnormal. He may make frenzied movements with his forelimbs rather than the usual stretching movements, as though he were panicking, convulsing or punching a punching bag. There may also be physical deformities, although this is a variable finding. Nevertheless, delivering the foal as quickly as possible with minimal trauma is the only way to maximize the chances of his recovery, and it is *essential* in order to protect the health and future productivity of the broodmare.

Identifying the problematic "behavior" is the first step in resolving this type of dystocia. In the case of the foal arching his neck, for example, the head will have to be directed out with enough pulling force to overcome the abnormal arching of the neck muscles. This is made difficult by the fact that there is little room to work in the birth canal and by the fact that the mare is usually straining valiantly, pressing your bruised arm into the bones of her pelvis while you attempt to grip the foal's muzzle with fingers that are rapidly getting numb from lack of circulation.

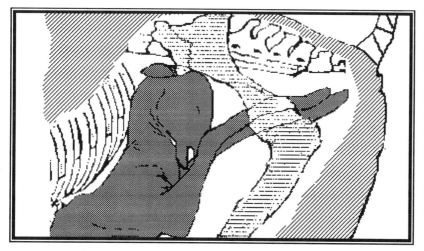

FIGURE 4.34
If the foal is arching his neck instead of extending it during delivery (usually an indication that something is wrong with him), his head will have to be directed out with enough pulling force to overcome the powerful abnormal flexing of his ventral (anterior, or front) neck muscles.

If at all possible, the foal's head should be directed by pulling with only the strength of the attendant's fingers, without the mechanical aid of "appliances" such as snares, hooks, chains or forceps. In some cases, however, the foal's jaw must be grasped by something stronger than tiring fingers, and a cable-type hog snare is usually most effective in getting a stronghold. This should only be used by a veterinarian, and only when the foal's condition is considered less important than the mare's, as it is almost certain to damage the foal. It is potentially dangerous to the mare as well, and the safety of her delicate tissues should always be considered with every insertion, every adjustment, every pull, every positional change—**every decision made in the process of resolving a dystocia should be made with the mare's safety foremost in mind.**

Once a firm grasp has been established on the foal's muzzle, traction can be applied to direct it into the birth canal. If the forelimbs have advanced (or been pulled) too far ahead of the foal's head, they should be gently but firmly pushed back in (repelled) while pulling on the head. This should help to make more room in the entrance to the birth canal. The head should be pulled until the foal's muzzle has reached the level of the "knees" (carpi) of the forelimbs, which is approximately normal delivery position. Then the head and both forelimbs, one about 6 inches ahead of the other, should be pulled simultaneously, being mindful of the arc-like pathway that the foal must follow in order to traverse the birth canal without rib and spinal damage.

FIGURE 4.35
Once a firm grasp has been established on the retained muzzle, traction should be applied to the muzzle without pulling on the forelimbs, which are already too far advanced. If necessary, the forelimbs can be pushed back in partially (repelled) while pulling on the muzzle in order to make room in the birth canal. Note that in this drawing the head is shown deflected to the side of the legs in order to minimize confusion.

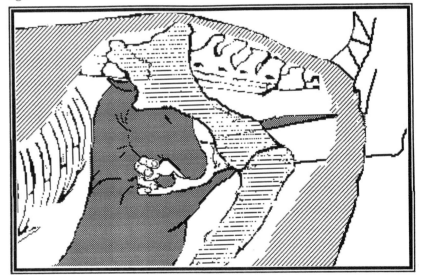

Overall, the vast majority of dystocias are fetal dystocias, meaning that they occur because the foal is, for one reason or another, positioned incorrectly. Maternal dystocia (the result of some problem with the mare rather than the foal) is much less common and more complicated to resolve, because the successful delivery of the foal will require much more than finding and straightening a folded leg.

The most common positional abnormalities in fetal dysto-cias involve the head and/or forelimb(s) of the foal. Only 1 in 500 deliveries involves "breech" (backwards) presentation of the foal. Although a deviation in the foal's position, per se, is not hazardous to his survival, it creates a life-and-death situation requiring quick action because of what happens during the labor process:

• The contractions of the uterus and of the mare's external abdominal muscles, which are powerful and progressive, will effectively push the malpositioned foal as far as possible into the birth canal before he becomes hopelessly wedged. If the con-tractions continue when movement of the foal through the birth canal is no longer possible, the foal and the tissues of the birth canal are subjected to intolerable pressure. Furthermore, any efforts to examine and correct the positional abnormality are hindered by the force of the contractions and by the potential for damage to the operator's arm when caught between the foal and the mare's pelvis during a contraction.

• After the onset of Stage II (i.e., after the water breaks), sep-aration of the placenta from the uterus begins to occur and continues progressively over time. As long as the mare's uterus is contracting, the survival of the fetus is increasingly threatened as more and more of the placenta detaches from the uterus, essen-tially choking off the oxygen supply to the fetus. After 30 to 40 minutes, there has often been sufficient separation to guarantee brain damage. Until the fetus is outside the mare, breathing his own oxygen and pumping his own blood, that placenta is his lifeline, and in order to function, the placenta must be plugged into the uterus as completely as possible. All living organisms can survive a certain amount of *oxygen* deprivation without suf-fering permanent damage, but deprivation of *blood* is another matter entirely, making the risk of serious and permanent dam-age a reality much sooner. Even the "normal" birthing creates a degree of oxygen deprivation (hypoxia), as evidenced by the fact that most foals turn a little blue during even the easiest deliv-eries. When *blood* deprivation (ischemia) occurs, however, the risk to the foal is almost immediate and more often leads to permanent damage or death. This is why the backwards ("breech") delivery is so dangerous to the foal—the umbilical

89

cord, which is the only route by which he receives the placental blood until the birthing is complete, is pinched sooner and more effectively between the weight of the foal and the mare's bony pelvis when the foal is in a backwards presentation. The foaling attendant should always bear in mind, therefore, that blood deprivation can occur by these two different means—by placental separation from the uterus, and by compression or pinching of the umbilical cord.

• The mare is also at risk during a dystocia. Obviously the tissues of the birth canal are in danger of being damaged, particularly when correcting the dystocia involves the use of "tools" and repeated manual manipulations, which increase the possibility of contamination and physical trauma to the vagina and cervix. Damage to these areas may delay or even prevent future reproduction. Of a more sinister and serious nature, however, is the risk of uterine rupture. The fluids that fill the placental "sacs" help to protect the mare as well as the fetus, but when the birthing process is prolonged for any reason, more and more of the fluids drain out, leading to uterine contracture around the fetus. Instead of supporting and heaving the foal out, cushioned by the volume of fluids, the uterus begins to *hug* the foal, eventually clinging to him like sandwich wrap. Normal protrusions of the foal, such as elbows, hocks, and hooves, now become potential trocars, able to poke through the tired and stretched tissues of the uterus and into the abdominal cavity. This is no longer merely a threat to the mare's reproductive future—it's a threat to her life. This is another reason to have the veterinarian on the scene and ready to act during all foalings—time is of the essence, and the mare must be protected. Which leads us to . . .

THE TWO COMMANDMENTS OF DYSTOCIA WORK

1. Thou shalt deal with the problem of straining

The biggest problem associated with dystocia is excessive straining on the part of the mare. There are several reasons why excessive straining needs to be remedied.

First, until the cause of the dystocia has been corrected, no amount of straining is likely to be successful in expelling the foal. The mare's intense efforts are serving only to exhaust her and to increase the risk of uterine and/or vaginal rupture and rectal and/or uterine prolapse.

Second, the malpositioned foal, which will not be able to fit through the birth canal in its current position, is becoming more tightly jammed in the canal with every push, making it more difficult to get your arm in there to figure out what the problem is and correct it.

Third, as we have already discussed, the chances of successfully correcting a positional abnormality and delivering a live, healthy foal become slimmer as time ticks by. The mare's expulsive efforts hinder your work, hurt your arm and delay the resolution of the problem.

Therefore, straining must be dealt with if faced with a serious dystocia. There are several tools and tricks that the veterinarian can employ to accomplish a dampening or deadening of the mare's contractions:

• **Pass a clean stomach tube into the mare's trachea (windpipe).** Since the abdominal press associated with straining requires a closed glottis (think about what you do with your throat when you strain), the ability to strain maximally will be hindered when the glottis is "propped" open by a skillfully placed stomach tube in the trachea. Under most other circumstances, the veterinarian usually tries to *avoid* placing the stomach tube in the trachea, since medications meant for the stomach would create disastrous results if deposited in the lungs, but in this one instance the tube is purposely placed down the "wrong" pipe. This is not necessarily easy to do, and it may take several tries before the tube is successfully directed into the trachea. It is made easier by holding the mare's head in an extended, stretched-out position. (By contrast, the head is flexed, nose to chest, to facilitate placing the tube into the "right" pipe, down the esophagus.) In minor dystocias, the veterinarian may find that the stomach tube in the trachea creates just enough of a reprieve from the straining to allow the dystocia to be corrected.

• **Administer short-term general anesthesia**. The decision to administer general anesthesia must be made with the mare's general condition in mind, since there is always an added element of risk when the patient is stressed and/or debilitated. In more complicated and/or advanced dystocias, however, the mare's straining reflex is so firmly entrenched and the power of the contractions is so overwhelming that the stomach tube in the trachea simply doesn't do enough. Although most mares will continue to strain while under the effects of short-term "field" anesthesia, the contractions are usually less powerful and the attendant is able to accomplish much more manipulation and repositioning of the foal. An added benefit is the fact that the anesthetized mare can be rolled over, rolled up onto her back and even hoisted or propped up in a position that helps the operator correct the abnormality. Bales of hay are invaluable in holding the anesthetized mare in position. The most popular field anesthetic currently (xylazine plus ketamine hydrochloride) will last for about 20 minutes, more or less, and usually provides for a smooth recovery, meaning that the mare remains recumbent until her legs are ready to support her, rather than flailing and struggling to get up while her legs are still rubbery.

• **Administer long-term general anesthesia.** This is usually reserved for the hospital setting, since the only safe way to keep a horse anesthetized for an extended period of time (an hour or more) is to use "gas" (inhalant) anesthesia with an electrically powered respirator and to support the mare's heavy body on specialized padded surfaces. Furthermore, most cases requiring long-term anesthesia are also candidates for surgery, and any abdominal surgery in horses, whether it be for a cesarean section or for colic, should be reserved for the controlled environment of a surgery room, since the horse is exquisitely sensitive to peritonitis (infection in the abdominal cavity) and postsurgical abdominal adhesions. Unlike the short-term anesthetic situation, uterine contractions cease when the mare is under long-term anesthesia, and the muscles of the uterus, abdomen and birth canal relax fully when the plane of anesthesia is deep. This provides for freer manipulation, unencumbered by muscle contractions and less restricted by space. The risk to the foal is far greater, however, since the effects of most drugs given to the mare will be directed to the foal as well. All these factors must be considered when selecting any drugs to be used in a dystocia.

• **Administer a low epidural nerve block ("spinal").** Many human obstetrical procedures are done with the patient "under a spinal," which leaves her awake and alert but feeling no pain. In equine obstetrics, the properly administered low epidural nerve block will eliminate straining while allowing the mare to have full use of her hind limbs. This makes it much easier to get your arm into the birth canal, since the muscles are relaxed and the mare is no longer responding to your manipulations with maximal straining. An added benefit is that epidurals do not adversely affect the foal. Remember, however, that the mare will no longer be able to provide as much *help* with the delivery by contracting and pushing maximally once the positional abnormality has been corrected. This is not an insurmountable problem, but it should be considered, especially if the mare is standing, since gravity works against the delivery of a foal from a standing mare that is not having uterine contractions. If the mare is recumbent, pulling the foal is less difficult.

The important points for the veterinarian to remember when administering the epidural is to choose the site of injection carefully and to choose the anesthetic agent and the dose injected with the specific needs of the case in mind. For most obstetrical purposes, a low epidural is given, whereby the injection is placed at the base of the tail, between the first two coccygeal (tail) vertebrae. The clinical difference between a low epidural and a high epidural, in terms of the effect on the mare, is that the high epidural nerve block interferes with the functioning of the mare's hind limbs. The high epidural results when the site of the injection is higher on the spine or when the dose of local anesthetic is increased so that the drug spreads farther forward and "numbs" more of the forward nerves in the spine, making it difficult or impossible for the mare to stand until the drug wears off. This may last for a relatively short time (30 minutes) or a very long time (12 hours or so), depending on the choice of drug and the dose given. Gravity also plays a role, and if the mare is lying down with her hindquarters elevated above her front end, the local anesthetic may simply flow forward and numb more of the forward spinal nerves. The properly administered low epidural nerve block dampens or eliminates uterine contractions, numbs the anus and vulva and the immediately surrounding area (the perineum) and has no effect on the function of the hind limbs. The best way to determine whether the low epidural has begun to take effect is to pinch or prick the lower edge of the mare's anus to see if it responds by "pursing." The anus will show no response if the nerve block has taken effect. Obviously this should not be attempted while in a vulnerable position, since a mare with full sensation in the anus may express her displeasure by kicking.

• **Administer other drugs to decrease straining.** Various degrees of success have been reported with the use of xylazine or detomidine, drugs that have marked sedative and pain-killing effects. Propantheline is reportedly very effective in halting uterine contractions for a short time (about 15 minutes) with virtually no sedative side effects, but it is not approved by the FDA for use in horses, and it is only available in the oral form for treatment of peptic ulcers in humans.

2. Thou shalt lubricate generously

The second biggest problem associated with dystocia is inadequate lubrication in the birth canal and in the uterus. Two things happen during the course of a dystocia that contribute to this problem.

First, the fluids that are initially gushing from the allantoic cavity of the placenta are running low and have, over time, rinsed away much of the more slippery mucus-like secretions in the birth canal. During the early stages of a normal birthing, the watery allantoic fluid mixes with the thick cervical and vaginal mucus to form a marvelous lubricant. After a little while, however, the mucus is rinsed away, leaving the soft tissues of the birth canal feeling "squeaky," actually *increasing* the friction between the foal and the mare.

Second, as more and more of the allantoic fluid is pushed out of the uterus during the mare's prolonged delivery attempts, the walls of the uterus begin to close in around the foal's body. This makes the contractions of the uterus much less effective in pushing the foal out. More importantly, however, it also makes the uterus much more vulnerable to tearing or rupture during contractions and during pulling of the foal by attendants. This is due to its closer proximity to elbows, hocks, hooves and other relatively sharp foal parts that are punching into the uterine wall if the foal is alive; it is also due to these same body parts being dragged against the tired, drying uterine walls when the foal is pulled.

Therefore, generous lubrication is warranted when dealing with a serious dystocia. Generous lubrication means pumping one or two gallons of suitable lubricant into the birth canal and into the uterus with a clean stomach tube and pump. Whenever needed, more lubricant should be added—lack of lubrication should *never* be allowed to become a factor in a failed delivery attempt. Adequate lubrication protects the mare's soft tissues against the ravages of the attendant's arm as well as the struggling foal, aids in the expulsion/traction of the foal, and may make all the difference in resolving a dystocia in time. Lubrication of the birth canal during a dystocia should not be considered a "maybe" or an optional luxury—it is an absolute necessity.

The choice of lubricant is important, since pumping foreign substances into the uterus may contribute to infection and/or direct damage to uterine tissue. The well-prepared equine veterinarian will carry several gallons of a suitable "lube" in the mobile vet unit, but *it is advisable for the mare owner to have a gallon or two in the foaling barn* just in case the veterinarian used all his lube at another call earlier in the day and didn't have time to restock before responding to the next call. The importance of good lubrication can't be overemphasized—don't let it be an oversight.

There are several obstetrical-grade lubricants available in the veterinary supply market that are sold in gallon quantities for pumping into the birth canal and uterus. If they are safe for intrauterine use, their labels will indicate as such. If the label does not mention intrauterine use, the product is probably *not* safe to use for anything except rectal palpations, either because the ingredients include antiseptics that can cause uterine inflammation, the product is not water soluble or it is not prepared in an aseptic (clean) environment.

Even when an approved, water-soluble, sterile lube is used, after the dystocia is resolved and the afterbirth is passed **the uterus should be flushed out repeatedly with sterile saline in order to facilitate the expulsion of any leftover fluids, lube and debris**. Whether or not the uterus should be infused with an antibiotic or antiseptic solution after the flushing is a judgment call for the veterinarian to make based on the characteristics of the individual case.

THE STANDING DELIVERY
Most mares will lie down to deliver. This is definitely the preferred position, since it's a long way down to the ground for the

foal to fall head first from a standing mare, and since such a fall would undoubtedly cause the immediate rupture of the umbilical cord and the loss of what appears to be a lot of blood. Some mares, however, will fail to lie down, usually because some external influence is disturbing their sense of security. In most cases, even the most nervous mares will eventually, *finally*, go down, but it is advisable to anticipate problems and make whatever changes may be necessary in your foaling environment ahead of time so that the mares will feel more at home there and will be more likely to lie down (see Section 3.5).

If your setup seems ideal and yet the mare still does not lie down, consider that human intervention is upsetting her. If there are too many people around, ask them to leave. If they are making too much noise, ask them to be quiet (or leave). And finally, consider that *you* should "disappear" as well. Back away until you are a reasonable distance away, preferably in the shadows or behind a wall, and be still and quiet. Most mares, even the most persistently nervous ones, will lie down during Stage II of labor if you give them enough privacy. If the mare approaches you in your hiding place, speak to her softly but remain still so that she knows it's you, not some sinister character, and you don't plan to interfere. Reassure yourself by remembering that you have already checked the position of the foal and everything is in place.

A delay of up to 20 minutes from the time the water breaks to the beginning of full labor contractions can be acceptable, especially if there are environmental factors that are distracting the mare. As long as the allantois-chorion has ruptured, the foal is probably still getting plenty of blood and oxygen through the umbilical cord. So stay put, and wait for the mare to lie down. If possible, allow her to deliver the foal completely by herself once she has gone down. But if it is necessary to help by providing a little traction on the foal during delivery, try not to approach the mare until she has been out flat for a few moments and has given a few obvious "pushes." Usually by this time she is engrossed in the labor process and is unlikely to care about your approach. However, try not to approach so slowly and stealthfully that you look like a stalking cat—this is the kind of thing horses are designed to be fearful of. Be quiet and respectful, but don't be sneaky. The mare knows you're there—what she doesn't know is whether or not you can be trusted during this time of crisis and vulnerability.

Sometimes a mare will actually wait until she has pushed the foal's forelimbs and head out before she finally lies down, so it would be wise to stay in your hiding place until absolutely the last minute, just in case she gives up and lies down. Otherwise, your approach may be just enough to convince her *not* to lie down. If you have done everything you can think of and the mare appears determined to deliver the foal while standing, you are left with no alternative but to go along with her misguided decision. Have your trusted, attentive partner hold the mare loosely at the head while you cradle the emerging foal in your waiting arms. The foal is heavy, wet, bloody, slippery and struggling, so it will take considerable strength and effort to support him. Try to hold him as close as possible to the mare's vulva so that the umbilical cord remains intact as long as possible, preferably at least 5 minutes. This is likely to require the strength of two people.

As soon as the umbilical cord ruptures, which should occur when you gently place the foal on the ground, treat the umbilical stump generously with your iodine solution, and check to make sure the stump is not bleeding. Have your assistant turn the mare around so that she can nuzzle the baby while you quickly tie up the placenta with the longer piece of cotton string from your pocket before the mare steps on the placenta and slips on it or tears part of it off.

A word of warning
Most mares are incredibly graceful when walking around a newborn foal, and even when the foal gets tangled up in the mare's legs and you're sure she's going to step on him, she deftly removes her legs from the tangle without a misstep. However, all natural grace and balance can disappear when humans are interfering, and even when you are performing necessary and vital tasks, some mares resent the human presence so much at this delicate time that they focus too much of their attention on worrying about what you're doing and forget about watching where they put their feet. **Be sure your assistant is paying attention to the *mare*, not the cute little foal.** Get your tasks accomplished and then get out of there.

Another word of warning

At this point, your remaining tasks will be the same as with a normal foaling, with the possible addition of slightly more risk that you'll be charged, bitten or kicked by the mare, since her refusal to lie down has already established that she's the nervous type, and most mares are exceptionally protective of their relatively helpless newborn foals during the first 24 to 48 hours after foaling. Even the sweetest mare can become suspicious and aggressive when she has a newborn foal to protect. Never assume that you are exempt from an attack or other aggressive behavior. **Be respectful of the mare's maternal instincts. Be careful!**

Section 4.6
Stage II, the Actual Delivery

It should be clear at this point that only the uninformed attendant will see the actual *delivery* of the foal as the "scary" part, since the drama of delivery is the only aspect of the foaling that they can see externally. If they had knowledge of what is happening on the inside of the mare prior to delivery, they would come to understand that real fortitude and courage are most crucial in the *earlier* stages, in predicting the time of foaling, in making sure the water breaks, and in checking for and correcting abnormalities in foal position. Once these steps have been taken, what remains is most likely to proceed without significant difficulty. It may be physically demanding, but in most cases the difficult judgments and decisions are behind you at this point. But if these steps are not understood, the false impression exists that the only task awaiting the foaling attendant is to "pull" the hapless foal. It is this same false impression that leads the uninformed to believe in the foaling alarm systems that sound the alert when the mare is actually expelling the foal. It should also be clear at this point that many foaling problems are going to be dangerously, irreversibly established by the time the alarm goes off, like a burglary that triggers the alarm as the thief is driving away.

THE STAGE II DILEMMA:
TO PULL OR NOT TO PULL?

In most cases pulling is not necessary and can cause unpleasant side effects if done too soon, too vigorously, too effectively or improperly. These conditions will be discussed later in this section. When warranted, however, judicious use of traction on the emerging foal can be helpful to the young, small or unconditioned mare that may become overly fatigued from a prolonged labor process. In the following section, the proper "pulling" technique will be discussed, as well as how to recognize when pulling is the *wrong* thing to do.

During the brief period of calm between the time when the water breaks and the uterine contractions actually begin, it is not uncommon to find that the front legs and nose of the foal are in a position that indicate that the foal is "upside down" in the mare. Since most reference publications on the foaling process state that the foal is in the "delivery position" days or even weeks before actually emerging from the mare, it could cause a bit of panic to find, when checking for position after the water breaks, that the foal is still upside down.

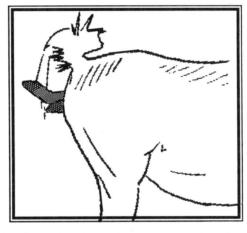

FIGURE 4.36
The soles of this foal's feet are facing the sky, indicating that the foal is still upside down. This is a common situation that usually resolves itself with little or no human intervention.

Don't panic—it's actually quite normal in most cases for the foal to be upside down at this stage—many of the old reference books are incorrect. In fact, the foal does not achieve the "delivery position" completely until it is already halfway out of the mare.

The contractions of the mare's uterus fall into two distinct categories: rotational and expulsive. The earliest contractions are rotational; i.e., they serve to roll the foal from his back over to one side and eventually onto his sternum. This is where the exercises that the foal was doing during Pre-Stage I become so very important, because now he is able to extend his neck and his forelimbs so that when the uterus rolls him over, his front

FIGURE 4.37
Normal foal position prior to the onset of Pre-Stage I.

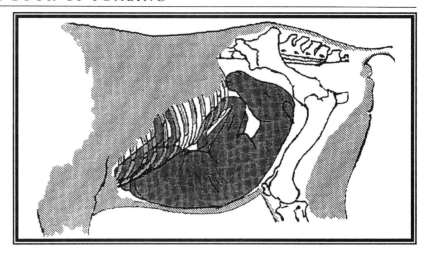

FIGURE 4.38 A,B
During Pre-Stage I, the foal makes purposeful movements in periods of high activity, then rests awhile before starting another flurry of activity. These movements, extending the neck and forelimbs, are "exercises" that prepare the foal for the active role he must play in positioning himself properly during the delivery.

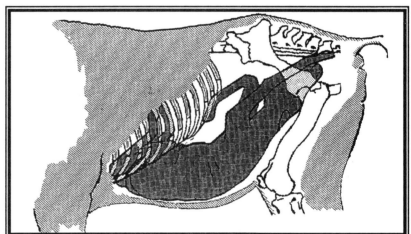

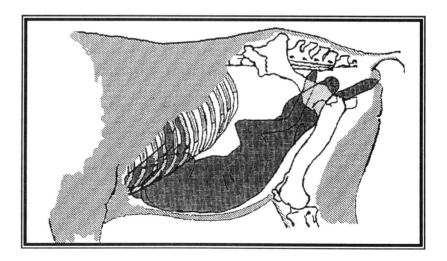

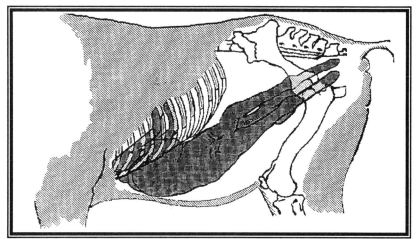

FIGURE 4.39
As Stage II begins, the rotational uterine contractions gradually begin to roll the front half of the foal over to one side.

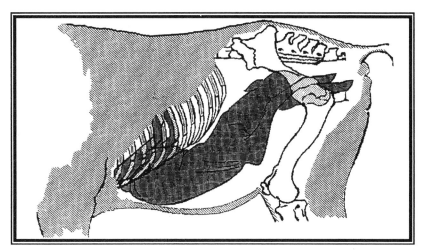

FIGURE 4.40
As the rotational contractions continue, the foal's front half eventually approaches the delivery position. Note that the foal's rear half is still passive and remains "upside down."

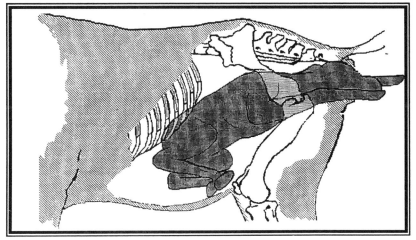

FIGURE 4.41
When the expulsive uterine contractions begin to push the foal through the birth canal, the foal's rear end passively flips over to follow the upright front end.

hooves and muzzle will extend into the mare's vagina. If the foal were not able to extend his neck and forelimbs and hold them in the extended position, one or more of these parts could return to the flexed position before the rolling process is complete, resulting in one of the abnormal positions discussed in Section 4.5, whereby one or more of the three essential parts is "missing."

A short while after the rotational contractions have begun, the expulsive contractions join in the process. The expulsive uterine contractions serve to push ("expel") the foal out. When the mare is obviously "pushing" from the outside, she is responding to expulsive uterine contractions on the inside, since the natural response to expulsive contractions of the uterus is to assist those contractions with a corresponding contraction ("push") of the external abdominal muscles. If the foal is still upside down during this stage, some mares may augment their rotational contractions with some rolling of their own in order to help the foal get rolled over into position. This is one of those situations where the old adage about never letting your horse roll over (for fear she'll "twist" something) may interfere with her attempts to position her emerging foal. In most cases, if the mare is allowed to correct the situation herself, she will repeatedly get up, turn around, lie back down, roll up onto her back abruptly once or twice, get up again, lie back down, roll some more and repeat the process for a minute or two until she has successfully repositioned the foal.

The problem comes in when the foaling attendant panics and tries to roll the foal over by sticking both arms in the mare's vagina and attempting to twist the foal. This could never be successful in rolling the foal, but more importantly, it will stimulate the mare's vagina and cause the expulsive contractions to occur sooner than they would ordinarily have occurred. If the expulsive contractions begin in earnest before the foal is adequately rotated, the odds of the foal becoming jammed in the birth canal are significantly increased. The key to success in dealing with an upside-down foal is to intervene only when absolutely necessary, and then to intervene in such a way as to rectify the foal's position without stimulating the mare's vagina and causing premature release of oxytocin and the resultant exacerbation of expulsive contractions.

It is essential to bear in mind that the mare has two kinds

of contractions and that the rotational contractions occur as a result of some hormonal influence other than oxytocin—probably prostaglandin. The delay between breaking water and the onset of expulsive contractions is likely due to a natural delay in the release of oxytocin, as though the body knows that the foal must be rotated before it can be expelled successfully, but any prolonged or vigorous stimulation of the mare's vaginal tissues during this natural lull can stimulate the premature release of oxytocin and result in expulsive contractions before the foal is properly positioned.

If the mare continues to exhibit the rolling behavior for more than a few minutes but is making no progress in rolling her foal, it may be necessary to assist her. It is very important to recognize that when the foal is upside down, he can poke a forelimb up through the mare's vagina and rectum if he remains upside down during expulsive contractions. In fact, it may be necessary to protect the roof of the mare's vagina and the floor of the rectum by repeatedly redirecting the foal's hooves until his position is corrected.

If it is decided that intervention is necessary to help the mare roll the foal, the first thing you should do is recheck the foal's position to make sure that there is not an extra leg in the birth canal. Make sure the mare's perineal area is clean before inserting your freshly gloved, lubricated hand. Once you have reassured yourself that exactly two forelimbs and one muzzle are present, try to assess whether the foal has tipped over to one side or the other. In other words, it's unlikely that the upside down foal is *perfectly* upside down; he will probably be leaning slightly to the left or to the right. This is important, because it will tell you in which direction the mare's uterus is trying to rotate the foal. It would be foolish for you to try to rotate the foal in the opposite direction, because you would be working against the efforts of the uterus.

If the foal is tipped to your left, the mare is trying to roll him over onto his left side. Grasp the foal's legs above the fetlock joint and cross the right leg over the left leg. Holding the legs crossed, wait for the mare to have a contraction (it will be more effective to do this if the mare is lying down), and while she pushes, you pull and twist, firmly but gently. This is not a procedure that should be done with more force than one person can apply. The addition of your assistance will permit the mare's rotational contractions to roll the foal—you will not be able to roll the foal without her help, and you should not try. Don't expect the foal to roll over abruptly—it will happen gradually, over the course of a few pushes. Do not pull while she is resting—pull only while the mare is pushing. It is permissible, however, to hold the foal "tense" in between the mare's pushes—i.e., to keep the foal from returning to the position it was in before the contraction. Do not lose sight of the fact that you are holding young, delicate, living limbs that will be damaged if you use excessive force.

FIGURE 4.42
If necessary, the foaling attendant can assist the process of rolling the foal over, but he must first determine which direction the mare's uterus is rotating. Otherwise the uterus may be working against the attendant's efforts. This foal is tipped to your left.

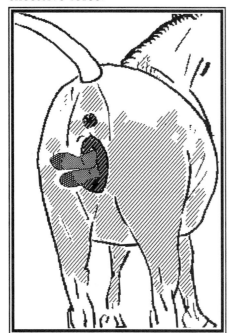

If the foal is tipped to your right, the mare is trying to roll him over onto his right side. Grasp the foal's legs above the fetlock joint and cross the left leg over the right leg and follow the same procedure as in the paragraph above.

Once the foal is rolled approximately into the correct position, it shouldn't be necessary for you to continue pulling—the mare should be able to finish the delivery alone. However, if the mare has been working hard and at least 10 minutes have passed since the contractions began, (and, most importantly, if the mare does not seem to mind your presence), it is permissible for you to provide a little assistance.

There are several good reasons it is not advisable to begin pulling too soon or too effectively. In other words, it is not necessarily good for a mare to deliver her foal after only a few minutes of contractions—oftentimes, the "easy" birthings are followed by long periods of significant colic-like discomfort in the mare called afterpains. Afterpains are hypothesized to be the result of uterine cramping when the uterus has retained a large volume of the fluids associated with the pregnancy. When the labor process lasts a little longer, the mare pushes significantly more of the fluids out before the foal emerges. Although uterine contractions continue to a degree after the foal is born, they tend to be less organized and less effective in expelling the retained fluids when the hard, heavy mass of the foal is no longer present.

The slightly skewed position of the foal's forelegs during birth is not an accident. It is essential that one leg be ahead of the other by approximately 3 to 6 inches, such that the tip of one hoof is approximately at the level of the fetlock of the other leg. This helps to reduce the overall width of the foal "package" that is advancing through the birth canal by situating one shoulder in the extended position and the other shoulder slightly flexed. If the forelegs are emerging at exactly the same level, then both shoulders will attempt to come through together in their widest position. This will prolong the delivery, increase the level and duration of pressure exerted upon the foal, increase risk of injury to the mare, increase risk of exhausting the mare and possibly deprive the foal of oxygen for a sufficient period of time to pose increased risk of damage due to lack of oxygen. If the forelegs are not adequately spaced, simply give one of them a gentle tug until the spacing is correct.

By the same token, it is important that the lead foreleg not be *too* far ahead of the trailing foreleg, because the trailing leg will begin to flex at the elbow if it gets too far behind. The flexed elbow is generally too bulky and may become lodged against the rim of the mare's pelvis ("elbow lock"), unable to enter the birth canal without significant damage to the foal and significantly increased effort by the mare, once more leading to a prolongation of the delivery process, increased pressure exerted upon the foal, possible oxygen deprivation and so on.

A good example of the hazards of elbow lock is offered by an emergency call I responded to in 1986. A mare was having difficulty expelling her healthy foal because one foreleg was slightly too far ahead of the other, and the well-meaning but ig-

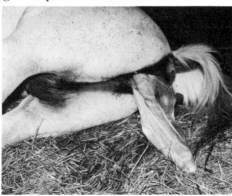

FIGURE 4.43
The tip of one hoof is approximately at the level of the fetlock of the other leg. Any deviation from this position, if the legs are even with each other or if they are too far apart, can lead to serious dystocia.

105

norant owner tried to help the mare by pulling only on the advanced foreleg. The harder the owner pulled, the more damage she did, because the trailing leg's elbow was now hopelessly lodged in the entrance to the birth canal in the fully flexed position. The leading leg was eventually pulled out all the way, giving the owner the mistaken impression that she was making progress. Her neighbor offered to help, and the two of them began to pull on the same extended leg. The hoof of the other foreleg remained uselessly within the mare's vulva, ignored by the mare's owner and her helper.

By this time the foal was weakening and beginning to fade away, so after a few minutes of fruitless pulling, the neighbor hooked the leading leg to a chain that was attached to the bumper of his Buick. The foal did not come out any further, despite the added power of the automobile, and by the time I was summoned to help, the foal was dead and the mare had been dragged across the pasture by the neighbor and his Buick, still tugging stupidly on the dead foal's foreleg. When I arrived, the neighbor took one look at my lightweight frame and spindly arms and shook his head, muttering something about obviously needing somebody with more strength. I walked up to the exhausted mare, gave the dead foal a firm push inward with one hand and reached the fingertips of my other hand just inside the lips of her vulva and gripped the hoof of the trailing leg, pulling it toward me with just the strength of my fingertips, thus straightening the elbow and positioning the leg so that it was just slightly behind the leading leg. The mare, sensing relief that the bulky elbow was no longer pushing against the rim of her pelvis, gave a little grunt and the dead foal slipped out onto the ground.

It is important at this point to envision the path that the foal must take in order to exit the uterus. During the last portion of the pregnancy, the foal is still forward of the birth canal, in the abdomen of the mare. In order to exit the mare, the foal must come up into the birth canal, go a short distance horizontally in the birth canal, and then aim slightly downward as it exits the birth canal. This is dictated by the shape of the birth canal, which is somewhat conical, narrower at the exit than at the entrance. The roof of the canal at the exit is formed by the first two coccygeal (tail) vertebrae, which are fused to each other and to the bony sacrum. The coccygeal vertebrae are slightly

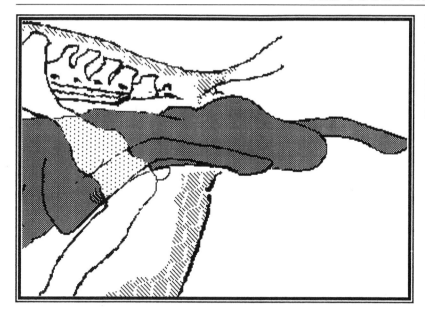

FIGURE 4.44
When one hoof is extended too far ahead of the other, the retained leg's elbow flexes and becomes lodged against the rim of the mare's pelvis.

angled in a downward direction, giving the roof of the birth canal a downward slope. If the foal tries to exit the birth canal "straight back," without angling downward, the roof of the birth canal will dig into his spine and the back of his chest as he emerges. **Overzealous and misdirected traction on the foal during delivery can force the foal through this narrowed portion of the birth canal at the wrong angle and cause serious damage to the delicate tissues of his thorax.** Foals that suffer fractured ribs and bruised lungs from such a delivery may seem normal at birth, but within two days their rapid breathing rate and deteriorated condition indicate internal damage, which is often too severe to allow veterinary intervention to save them.

It is essential that any traction be applied *only* while the mare is pushing. To understand the reason for this, imagine that you are standing in front of a closed, locked door on a loose rug that lies on a tile floor. What will happen to the rug if you grasp the door knob and pull on it as hard as you can? Since the door is locked, your efforts will pull you toward the door, and the rug will slip across the tile, bunching up between the door and your feet. This is similar to what happens to the tissues of the mare's vagina and uterus if you pull on the foal when the mare is not pushing. Although the goal of your efforts is to pull the foal through the canal, part of the canal will simply bunch up if you

107

FIGURE 4.45
The birth canal is cone-shaped due to the downward slope of its "roof." In order to navigate this pathway without injury, the foal must travel up from the abdomen, across the birth canal, and down to exit. The trip should be viewed as an arc.

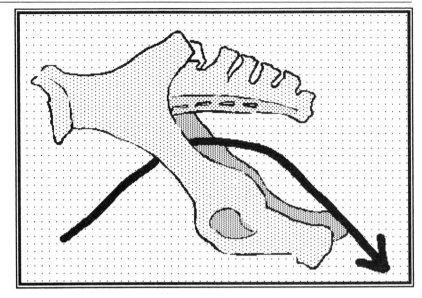

FIGURE 4.46
Pulling a foal in the manner illustrated here can result in serious, even fatal, damage to his ribs, lungs and/or spine. As in this example, the incorrect direction of pull can force the foal's body against the ceiling or floor of the mare's bony pelvic canal.

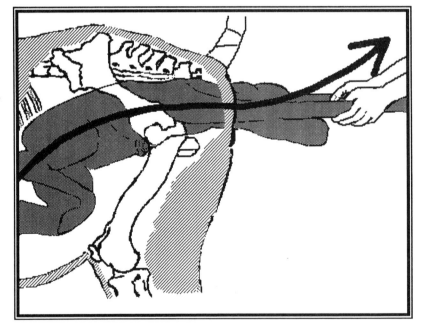

pull when the mare is not pushing. This not only fails to pull the foal out, it also serves to make it more difficult to get the foal out, since the bunched-up tissue of the birth canal is essentially making it more crowded in there. Furthermore, the friction that naturally exists between the foal and the canal can actually lead to tearing of the canal's tissues as well as the uterus itself if your untimely traction is forceful enough (see information on lubrication in Section 4.5). It is not uncommon, when responding to

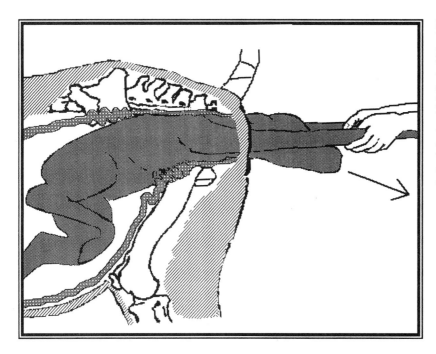

FIGURE 4.47
When the mare is not pushing, any attempts to pull the foal are likely to result in a "bunching up" of the soft tissues lining the birth canal. This crowds the birth canal, making it more difficult for the foal to fit through, and it also increases the risk of damage to the mare.

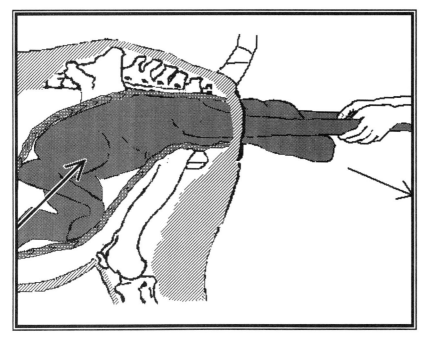

FIGURE 4.48
Traction applied while the mare is pushing is more likely to result in progress.

an emergency foaling call, for a veterinarian to find a live but traumatized newborn foal lying next to a mare that is in shock and probably dying because the attendants panicked and pulled too hard, too soon, when the mare was not pushing, resulting in a ruptured uterus. **Always remember that pulling at the wrong time and when the birth canal and uterus are inadequately lubricated can lead to serious damage to the mare's soft tissues.** The mare's future as a broodmare (and, in fact, her life) may hang in the balance.

The emerging foal is usually still encased in the filmy, milky-white sac called the amnion, and there is some controversy as to when (or whether) it should be ripped open by the foaling attendant. In unassisted foalings, the amnion usually rips open by itself on the foal's front hooves when his shoulders emerge from the mare, since the sac is usually stretched tightly over the leading hoof at that point in the delivery. The foal's tendency to stretch his forelimbs ahead of him during the final phase of the delivery may be a natural process designed to poke through the amnionic sac. Failure of the amnionic sac to tear has often been blamed for death by suffocation of the foal when unattended foalings occur and the owner finds the dead foal still encased in the intact sac. Although a number of other possibilities could have caused the foal's death, the failure to attend the foaling makes it impossible to know with any degree of certainty whether the foal would have survived if someone had been there to open the sac.

The moment when the foal takes his first breath is not known, as there are many factors that can affect the length and difficulty of the labor process as well as the forces brought to bear on the foal. Most researchers agree that when the concentration of carbon dioxide in the bloodstream reaches a certain level, signaling that oxygen is needed, the respiratory center in the brain stimulates the muscular diaphragm to move and the chest to expand, attempting to fill the lungs with air. Whether or not other factors influence this system is not known, but it has been suggested that the tension on the umbilical cord, the release of pressure on the foal's chest as it emerges from the birth canal, postural changes in the foal's position with respect to the mare and the stress of the delivery process in general are possible stimuli for the foal to gasp. It is a system that can fail in several instances, and it seems reasonable that more than one factor plays a role in governing the timing of the foal's first breath.

For example, most foals will actually begin to turn blue (become cyanotic) to varying degrees during the birthing, particularly if the delivery process is slightly prolonged or if the foal is an especially tight fit through the birth canal. If excessive carbon dioxide (and too little oxygen) are the *only* factors that stimulate breathing, many foals would gasp their first breath while still encased in the amnion, possibly inhaling particulate matter and meconium (foal's first manure) into their lungs. In truth, this does occur sometimes, and the consequences are serious. But the low frequency of cases that take their first breath too soon, when the risk of inhaling manure and other waste material is high, does not correlate well with the high frequency of cases that turn blue during the delivery, since the majority of foals undergo this "oxygen panic" but apparently manage to hold their breath until it's safe to inhale. Nevertheless, since the potential exists for the foal to inhale dangerous substances into his lungs during the birthing, it is recommended to **rip the amnion open as soon as the foal's muzzle emerges from the mare's vulva**. Clear all amnionic tissue away from the foal's nostrils and "strip" the nostrils of any liquid or solid material by firmly pinching and stroking the top of his face, from beneath his eyes to the tip of his nose, several times in the downward direction only. This not only serves to clear out the nostrils, it is also somewhat stimulatory to the foal and may help to get the breathing process started. Meanwhile, the mare is in the throes of labor and is exerting incredible force on the foal in her attempt to finish expelling him from her womb. This is the most critical time during the normal foaling, since the physical stress on the foal is at its peak at the same time that he is beginning to make delicate adjustments to sustain himself on the outside. If something goes wrong at this stage, the foal may fade away and die before the delivery is complete.

If, for example, all factors combine to tell the foal to inhale, but he is still wedged in the mare's birth canal and can't expand his chest to breathe because it is compressed in the canal, his oxygen debt will rise over the critical level, resulting in permanent brain damage. All living beings can survive a certain amount of oxygen deprivation without suffering permanent damage, but the danger zone is not far beyond. It is expected that the foal may begin to turn blue during the normal foaling, but steps should be taken at that point to abbreviate the delivery process so that the foal is not without oxygen any longer than absolutely necessary.

By the same token, the placenta is continuing to detach from the uterus, bit by bit, during the maximal contractions of Stage II. This means that the foal is receiving less and less oxygen from the mare, and he is not only at risk of inadequate oxygen (hypoxia)—he's actually at risk of receiving *no* oxygen (anoxia). And if the oxygen debt is severe enough to affect his heart, it can lead to general shutdown in circulation and blood deprivation (ischemia). Consider the underwater swimmer: he can frog-kick to his heart's content without breathing for over a minute, and as long as he doesn't inhale any water, he will recover with full brain function even after passing out, deprived of oxygen for a few minutes more. Now consider a victim of strangulation in a murder movie—the strangler overcomes his victim by shutting off the blood flow to the brain (the carotid arteries), and death occurs much more quickly than if the victim were merely deprived of oxygen. With these examples in mind, return now to the distressed foal: if ever there was a time for you to pull, the time is now.

Remember to pull in the proper direction with respect to the foal's progress through the arc-like pathway he must follow. Remember also to consider his delicate legs and the damage you can do to them if you pull improperly. Remember to pull only when the mare is pushing, and if she is not pushing enough during this critical time, stimulate her to do so by moving the foal's legs within the vagina. Once the foal's neck has begun to emerge, you can transfer your grip by grasping a handful of mane and the crest of the neck at the base of the mane, as close to the withers as possible, since this additional grip will be more effective in directing the foal through the canal properly. At no time should you lose sight of the fact that you are pulling on live tissues that can be damaged if your efforts are too vigorous and/or not properly directed.

In most cases, once the shoulders have cleared the birth canal, the delivery is essentially completed. Occasionally, however, one edge of the foal's pelvis becomes hooked on the edge of the mare's pelvis, bone against bone, in a dangerous situation called "hiplock." Even though most of the foal's body has emerged from the mare and is in the clear, the locked pelvises hold the foal in a position that places him at significant risk of oxygen deprivation, since his

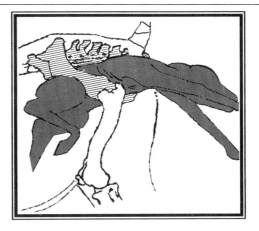

FIGURE 4.49
When the foal's pelvis is hooked on the rim of the mare's pelvis ("hiplock"), the foal is held in a location that restricts his chest and makes it impossible for him to breathe, even if his head is outside the mare.

umbilical cord is pinned between his weight and the mare's pelvic brim, and he is not yet able to breathe enough air into his own chest to avoid suffocation.

The reason hiplock occurs relates to the continuously changing position of the foal during delivery. Remember that the foal starts upside down, on his back. The mare's first contractions, which are rotational, begin to roll him over to one side. Meanwhile, he has extended his head and forelimbs so that they enter the birth canal in the extended position as he is rolling over. The rotational contractions continue along with the addition of the expulsive contractions, rolling the foal gradually into the "delivery position" as he emerges. Usually by the time his chest emerges from the birth canal, his hips and rear limbs are able to "flip" over to follow the chest's lead with no difficulty. However, if the mare has an expulsive contraction just at the time when the foal's pelvis is in the process of rolling over into the delivery position, the foal's pelvis can be just at the right angle to get hung up on the edge of the mare's pelvis when the mare's expulsive contraction pushes the foal's pelvis against the protruding rim of her own pelvis.

Hiplock is easy to correct and requires no more than the strength of one person. It is helpful to realize that the problem is *not* that the foal's pelvis is too *large*, it is simply lodged at one side, much like a wheelbarrow that easily fits in an alleyway, but as you push it into the entrance of the alleyway from an angle, you cut the corner a little too closely and get one edge of the wheelbarrow hung up on the edge of the wall.

To correct hiplock, grasp the foal's legs firmly with both

hands and pull the foal down and to the left, then down and to the right, then down and to the left again, and so on until you have "walked" the foal's pelvis through the mare's pelvis, much the same way you would "walk" a heavy appliance across a kitchen floor. The alternating sideways direction of your downward pull dislodges the locked edges and permits the delivery to continue.

Occasionally a delivery will seem to be progressing normally—the water breaks, the foal's position is checked and found to be normal, and the mare lies down, but then little or no progress is made because suddenly the mare seems disinterested in pushing. She may even get up and resume grazing, as though the foaling process never started.

There are two aspects to the expulsive efforts of the mare— one is involuntary and one is (to a degree) voluntary. The involuntary portion involves the actual contractions of the uterus, and the voluntary portion involves the purposeful "pushing" by the mare's external abdominal muscles, which are designed to augment the uterine contractions. As a rule, the external abdominal muscles will push when "cued" by the uterine contractions.

A lack of uterine contractions is a condition called uterine inertia. There are several reasons why this may occur, depending upon how long the mare remains content to "forget" about delivering her foal. The most common situation is actually not uterine inertia at all, occurring normally as a *temporary* reprieve from the stretching and discomfort of Stage I. Since the cervix should be completely dilated by this time, and the breaking of the water has allowed much of the fluid to be expelled, there is a significant reduction in the intrauterine pressure. Some mares appear to have so much relief from pain at this point that the discomfort that remains is almost unnoticeable, and they temporarily seem to "disconnect" from the activities taking place within the uterus. Usually the movement of the foal within the birth canal stimulates the beginning of serious contractions, the same way that the presence of the foaling attendant's arm in the vagina during the foal position examination often has a stimulatory effect, bringing the contractions on sooner than if the examination had not taken place.

By the same token, however, if the foal is *not active enough* within the birth canal, there may not be adequate stimulation to bring the mare into contractions. It is advisable, therefore, to give some attention to whether the foal is moving when checking for foal position. In most cases the foal is quite active, pulling his legs back a short distance, then stretching them out. Occasionally the activity of the foal is decreased or delayed, as though the foal were weak or asleep, and giving one leg a little push or pull (or both) with your hand is sufficient to get the foal moving. This benign intervention will also provide some stimulation for the mare, and oftentimes she will begin contractions after having the foal's legs manipulated.

If manipulating the foal's legs produces no "pushing" response on the mare's part, it may be necessary to stimulate the birth canal further by inserting your arm alongside the foal into the mare's vagina.

Remember that with each successive invasion into the birth canal, the threat of contaminating the mare's tissues and creating a reproductive tract infection is intensified. If it isn't necessary to invade, don't. If it seems necessary, be sure to do it cleanly. Don't get sloppy. This means, once again, that the mare's tail wrap should be repaired if any upper tail hairs have worked their way loose, the tail should be tied casually off to the right side and the mare's vulvar area should be washed again using your mild soap solution, clean warm water and clean wads of cotton. Do it thoroughly but quickly.

Wearing a fresh sterile shoulder glove coated with sterile lube, press your fingers together to flatten your hand, hold it upright in the handshake position and glide it gently into the vagina along one side of the foal. In most cases the mare will begin straining immediately and the birthing will continue. If not, take this opportunity to examine foal position again, paying particular attention to whether any extra parts are present. Check the rim of the pelvis for one or two extra hooves, since occasionally a rear hoof can get lodged there if the foal's rear limbs were flexed up against his midsection when the mare's rotational contractions turned him over. If no positional abnormalities are found and the mare is still not making any effort to expel the foal, check again for signs of life in the foal. If the foal is alive, all efforts should concentrate on getting the mare to push him out as soon as possible.

115

Remember this extremely important point: **it is highly un-likely that a foal would survive being pulled out if the mare isn't pushing**. In other words, if the foal is alive and the mare seems disinterested in pushing, grabbing the foal's legs and pull-ing is not necessarily the best course of action. First, such an action could be injurious to the mare's birth canal and causes the soft tissues lining the canal to "bunch up" ahead of the foal, making his pathway even smaller and tighter. Furthermore, if you are able to pull the foal only partway before he becomes lodged in the canal, you may be leaving him in a position where it is even more difficult for him to survive. Within reason, as long as he remains within the broad expanses of the mare's abdomen, he is at much less risk than if he were in the hard, narrow, pinched confines of the birth canal.

At this stage, for the sake of the foal, your veterinarian should focus his or her attention on the mare to determine why she isn't making expulsive efforts. Many factors could be causing her lack of response, including nutrition (e.g., inadequate cal-cium, inadequate energy, or overall poor health), hormone imbalance or deficiency (e.g., inadequate oxytocin and/or inad-equate response to oxytocin), fetal factors (e.g., if the fetus is deformed or otherwise abnormal and is not providing the proper cues for the mare's labor system) or just plain exhaustion (e.g., if she hasn't the endurance to continue trying). If it is deter-mined that the mare will be unable to provide adequate assis-tance for a normal pelvic delivery, the decision should be made *now* whether to opt for surgery (cesarean section) or assisted pelvic delivery. If the latter approach is elected but fails to extract the foal, the mare and foal may be sufficiently weakened by this time to be very poor surgical candidates. In other words, abdominal surgery in horses is always a gamble, but if the patient is already in compromised condition when entering the surgery room, the risks may have become unacceptably high. The ex-pense is also a major consideration. Your surgical dollars are best spent if all attempts are made to maximize the odds of survival for mare and foal.

If the pelvic delivery assistance approach is elected, the veterinarian will have several options, depending on the circum-stances. If the mare is in any way impeding the extraction by struggling or wearing herself out by straining inappropriately, the veterinarian may opt to anesthetize her. Of course this eliminates any assistance the mare could give in the delivery, but it also provides the opportunity to position her to best advantage by situating her on a hillside or by hoisting her front half skillfully with a block and tackle so that the aid of gravity

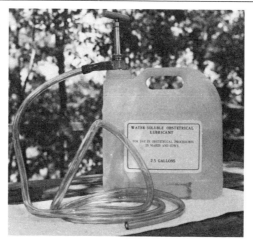

FIGURE 4.50
When attempting to pull a foal during a dystocia, the generous use of water-soluble obstetrical lubricant is essential. As much as two gallons of lube is pumped into the birth canal using a clean stomach tube and a hand pump.

can be enlisted. Whether the assisted pelvic delivery is attempted with the mare standing or under anesthesia, the pelvic canal should be generously lubricated with at least a gallon of water-soluble obstetrical lubricant. Most veterinarians who attend equine birthings carry large volumes of "lube" and can administer it into the birth canal using a clean stomach tube and hand pump.

Without the use of additional lubricant, and if the delay is permitted to persist for too long, the birth fluids that naturally lubricate the birth canal will eventually stop flowing, the birth canal will become overly dry and the delivery will be very difficult due to lack of lubrication, even if the mare's uterus is responding to your intervention by pushing. This is a common sequela to stillbirths and is often misinterpreted to be a situation in which the mare had a "difficult birthing" that caused the death of the foal. Actually, in many cases it's the other way around—the foal was already dead, and this caused the difficult birthing because the lack of movement of the dead foal allowed the mare's uterus to "go to sleep" instead of expelling the foal. This is the type of situation that occurs most commonly when the owner misses the foaling and finds the mare chewing contentedly on her hay while the forelimbs of the dead foal protrude from her unlubricated vulva.

Resolving the situation involves lubricating the birth canal and uterus generously with clean, water-soluble lubricant, then attempting to "awaken" the mare's uterus into cooperating while traction is applied simultaneously from the outside. This kind of delivery is often very difficult, despite the fact that the foal is not

117

oversized or lodged in any way, because the lack of lubrication causes increased friction with the birth canal, and the mare's uterus is not hormonally "primed" to participate in the delivery. In some cases general anesthesia of the mare makes it easier to pull the foal even though it eliminates the possibility of getting help from the mare, because it causes relaxation of the muscles around the vagina and vulva, and because the anesthetized mare is in the horizontal position, eliminating the need to work against gravity and pull the foal up out of the abdomen. It may be helpful to position the anesthetized mare such that her hindquarters are downhill, thereby eliciting the aid of gravity in getting the foal out. Since the mare is not pushing, and since the birth canal may be inadequately lubricated, the risk of tearing the uterus and/or vagina during such a delivery is significantly increased. For this reason, **extraction of a dead foal should never be undertaken without a veterinarian.**

On the other hand, if you are already there when the birthing of the dead foal starts (rather than trying to resolve an already dried-up birthing problem), you may be able to stimulate the mare to deliver the dead foal "normally" by manipulating his legs, gently but definitely moving them in and out, one leg at a time, the way a live foal would move. Nevertheless, veterinary attention should be considered mandatory to try to determine the cause of the foal's death and to ascertain whether any corrective measures need to be taken on the mare's behalf (such as treatment for a diagnosed uterine infection, for example).

In most cases, however, the foal is alive and struggling during the birthing, already preparing to adjust to his new tasks of breathing and pumping his own blood. If the foal seems too weak and does not appear to be breathing, strip out his nostrils again by vigorously stroking the top of this face with your hand in a downward, eyes-to-tip-of-nose direction. At the same time, open his mouth and clear it of any foreign material and give a gentle but definite tug on the tongue. If no response follows, slap him soundly on the side of his chest a couple of times with the palm of your open hand and shake him vigorously for a few moments, as though you were trying to awaken him from a sound sleep. A vigorous rubbing with a terrycloth towel may also stimulate him.

If you are still getting no response, and if you have the

strength to do this, pick the foal up and hang him upside down by holding him in a bear hug with your arms around his mid-section just ahead of his rear legs. Naturally the umbilical cord will have to be separated in order to do this. Holding the foal in this manner, try to turn around and around, spinning the foal around the axis of your body, to loosen and dislodge any material that may be blocking his airway. Place the foal gently back on the ground and try to ascertain if his heart is beating by grasping the lower edge of his chest behind his elbows with one hand. If the heart is beating but there is still no breathing response, mouth-to-nose resuscitation will be necessary until your veterinarian arrives with an emergency oxygen setup. Placement of a small dose of the respiratory stimulant doxapram hydrochloride under the foal's tongue, or injection of the drug into his umbilical vein or artery by the veterinarian occasionally succeeds as a last-ditch effort to start spontaneous breathing. If the heart is not beating, you will also have to try to stimulate the heart.

CPR

CPR (cardiopulmonary resuscitation) in the newborn foal is very similar to CPR in the adult human. However, a newborn's chest wall is not as rigid as an adult human's, and the heart and lungs are not as protected as you might expect. The idea of CPR is to massage the heart into pumping blood until it gets organized to do it alone, and to inflate the lungs with air to keep things going until respiration occurs spontaneously. Realistically, if the foal's heart is not beating, your chances of resuscitating him are slim. If his heart is beating, your chances of resuscitating him are better, depending on how traumatized he is and how soon you get to work. Recheck his mouth for foreign material and clear it if necessary. With the foal lying on his right side, close his mouth and pinch the lower nostril with one hand, then place your lips over his upper nostril and blow an average lungful of your air into his nostril until you see his chest rise. Then remove your lips and allow the air to escape. Repeat this process again and again, giving the foal approximately one breath every three seconds. If heart resuscitation is also necessary, a second person will be needed to apply quick, firm nudges to the heart with the heel of the hand on the foal's chest just behind the elbow on the foal's left side. Remember that the idea here is to massage the heart, not to bruise it or crack a rib. Your external efforts should create an artificial heartbeat once every second. If a few minutes have passed and your resuscitative efforts have produced no results, it would probably be wise to admit defeat and quit, because even if the foal were to revive at this point, it is highly unlikely that he would be free of brain damage and survive for more than a few hours.

Happily, in most cases the foal is strong and able to adjust and breathe normally after the birthing ordeal. Once the foal's hips have cleared the birth canal, the mare will usually lie quietly and rest, apparently unconcerned with her foal for a few moments, until the "fog" clears from her head and she regains her strength.

UMBILICAL CORD

Most foaling texts recommend that the umbilical cord be protected from rupture until 10 minutes after the foal has emerged. This requires that every effort be made to minimize the noise and activity around the mare and foal so as not to "awaken" the mare from her "hypnotic" post-foaling state too soon, since the cord will rupture when the mare stands. Time seems to tick by

FIGURE 4.51
Once the foal's hips have cleared the birth canal, the mare usually will lie quietly for several minutes until the "fog" clears from her head.

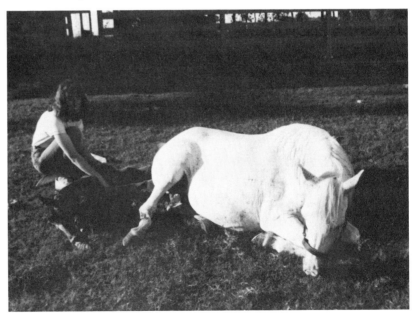

extremely slowly at this stage, so you should try to get into the habit of looking at your watch as soon as the foal emerges so that you will know how long the umbilical cord has remained intact.

With very few exceptions, **the umbilical cord should be allowed to rupture on its own,** that is, it should not be cut or ripped by human attendants, since the odds of bleeding and contamination are increased with such intervention. One exception would be if the mare passes the afterbirth while the umbilical cord is still intact. Similarly, if the mare is very weak

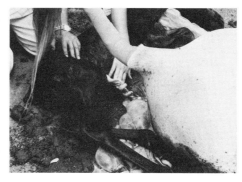

FIGURE 4.52
The umbilical cord was designed to separate at a predetermined place about one inch from the foal's abdomen. It is not uncommon, by the way, for the umbilical cord to be quite twisted, as in the example in this photograph.

and is unable to rise for a long while after foaling, manually stretch and break the cord at its predetermined breaking point after 15 or 20 minutes. Cutting it with scissors or a knife is not advised, since the stump will almost always bleed and must be tied off, leaving it vulnerable to infection.

Unless the foal is very active, his rear legs often remain within the mare's vagina until the mare stands or an attendant removes them. Oddly enough, it seems that the mare is more likely to be disturbed and stand prematurely if the foal's feet are not in her vagina. Therefore, unless the foal is being unnecessarily rough on the mare's vagina and you fear that she will be damaged by leaving them in, do not remove them.

In order to keep the situation as relaxed as possible, only one or two people should be attending the mare and foal at this point. If your knowledge of the mare's disposition suggests that a person at her head would serve to keep her from standing too soon, then the person who handled the mare's head throughout the foaling should remain with her, crouched down and as non-verbal and unobtrusive as possible. Both attendants should refrain from speaking to the mare or patting her "reassuringly," since this would only attract her attention to your presence and possibly arouse her too soon. Do not speak to each other, light a cigarette, open a can of pop, scratch an itch, cough, sneeze or in any other way draw attention to yourself if at all possible. Try to be invisible. Furthermore, if your observations and/or your knowledge of the mare's disposition suggest that she would be more likely to stay down if the person at her head "disappeared," quietly indicate as such to your assistant. Don't allow observers to conceal themselves behind the mare where she would have to get up and turn around to see them—her ability to sense their presence should not be underestimated, and if she feels the need to assess them visually in order to determine whether or not they are a threat, she'll get up.

Be prepared for this portion of the foaling process by discussing ahead of time the possible course of the foaling, your tentative plans in each case and the unobtrusive and sensitive manner in which any movements should take place, paying attention to the noise of footsteps, clanging chains at gate latches, creaking hinges, etc. Leave the dog in the house or otherwise confined so that there will not be any sudden scurries or barking if a cat or mouse or some other "dangerous" intruder should happen to pass by and tempt the dog to give chase. Furthermore, dogs are attracted to the smells associated with foaling and may not be able to resist the temptation to sniff around, which could be quite unnerving for the mare.

The designated foaling attendant should remain crouched at the mare's rear, quietly ready with the bottle of iodine and the short piece of cotton string to sanitize the fresh umbilical stump and to tie if off *if and only if* it bleeds persistently after breaking. If you had not had the foresight to carry these items with you in your pocket, it would be necessary for you to walk over to your foaling basket now to get them, once again running the risk of disturbing the mare.

Although it is also important not to disturb the foal too much, *his* movements seem to be less disturbing to the mare than human movements, even if he is bumping her or knocking her with his awkward little legs. Therefore, it is permissible to perform certain routines on the foal if necessary while you are there, as long as you can be quiet and relatively unobtrusive.

For example, the foal's lungs contain a rather large volume of clear liquid, which must be expelled during the early hours of his life in order to make the lungs more effective air exchangers and to prevent opportunistic infectious organisms ("germs") from becoming established in the fluid and causing pneumonia. These fluids are more likely to remain in the lungs and accumu-

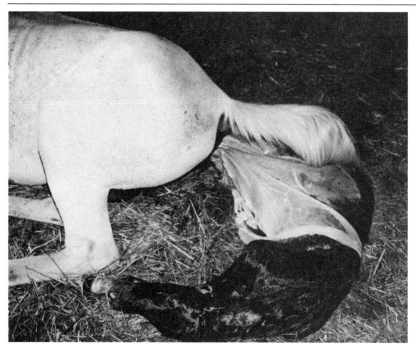

FIGURE 4.53
Often the mare and her newborn foal will rest quietly while the foal's rear legs remain in the mare's vagina.

late there if the foal lies flat out on his side for too long. If the surface the foal is lying upon is not level, and/or if he is fatigued or weak, it may be difficult for him to rise to the upright position on his sternum. With very little effort, you can pull the foal to the sternal position and, if necessary, prop him up against your

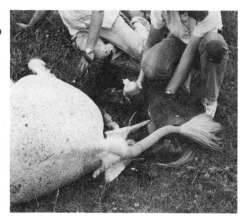

FIGURE 4.54
The primary foaling attendant remains quietly crouched at the mare's rear until the umbilical cord is ruptured by movement of the mare and/or foal. The bottle of surgical iodine solution is in hand, ready to disinfect the fresh stump.

crouched body so that he can get accustomed to supporting himself in this position. Sometimes an ounce or more of the clear liquid will drizzle steadily from his nostrils while he experiments with his newfound abilities to breathe and balance on his own.

The anatomy of the lungs is similar to the structure of a sponge, made up of tiny chambers called alveoli, which are collapsed at first but which inflate when the foal takes his first few

123

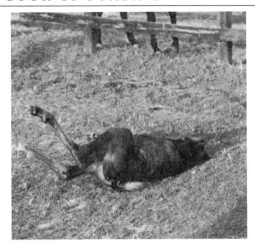

breaths of air. Oftentimes the alveoli situated in the farthest reaches of the lungs are the last to drain out the fluid completely and fill with air, and the fluid that remains can hold the walls of the tiny alveoli together in the collapsed position. Most veterinarians agree that the foal's clumsy attempts to stand up and walk during the next hour, which are almost always accompanied by some spectacular nosedives, are part of nature's system to "slap" the remaining fluid out of the lungs and fill the most peripheral alveoli with air when the foal gasps upon impact with the ground. Since it would be impossible for the mare to hold her newborn foal upside down by his rear legs and slap his bottomside the way some obstetricians handle newborn humans, it stands to reason that nature found a way to get the newborn foal to accomplish the same goal himself.

The umbilical cord emerges from the central "seam" of the foal's abdomen in a region that was left "unstitched" in order to permit the umbilical artery and veins to traverse the opening and provide blood flow to and from the foal. This is an inherent weak spot in the abdomen that can be the site of an umbilical hernia if the "unstitched" portion is larger than necessary, permitting some of the abdominal contents to protrude. In many cases umbilical hernias are the result of a mistake in the final developmental stages of foal growth in the mare; that is, the tendency to have an umbilical hernia is inherited from the genetic makeup of the ancestors. This presents the breeder of such an animal with the heavy responsibility of deciding whether it is advisable to continue breeding animals that are predisposed to such a defect. Umbilical hernias are rather simple and straightforward to repair surgically, but it would be unfair and unethical to have an umbilical hernia repaired and then sell the animal as a breeding prospect without informing the buyer that the defect existed.

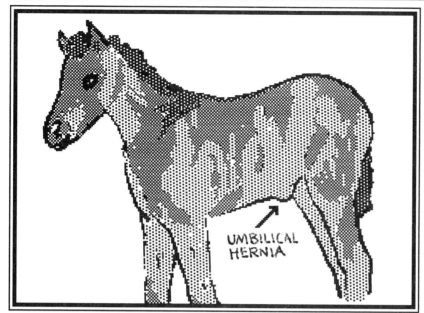

FIGURE 4.56
An umbilical hernia occurs when the central "seam" of the foal's abdomen has an opening in it that allows some of the abdominal contents to slip through the opening into the space under the skin and surface tissues.

In some cases, however, an umbilical hernia can be acquired rather than inherited, and careful attention to this possibility during the foaling can prevent an acquired herniation from occurring. We have already established that the umbilical region is potentially weak at first, since it is a natural and necessary hole in the seam of the foal's ventral abdomen. In the normal situation, the hole gradually heals closed during a period of several days to a few weeks after the cord breaks. The umbilical cord is designed to break at a predetermined spot, essentially a "dotted line" situated approximately an inch to an inch and a half from the foal's abdomen. The cord breaks when subjected to a moderate amount of tension shortly after birth due to the gradual or abrupt separation of mare and foal as they move around while still recumbent or when one of them suddenly stands up. However, in some cases the cord is reluctant to break, and it is subjected to excessive tension before it finally ruptures. This excessive tension on the umbilical cord causes an exceptionally hard pull on the abdominal wall of the foal, and it is possible that the normal, small opening in the abdomen can be "ripped" into a larger hole, essentially creating a hernia that was not there at birth. Although the controversy may exist that a perfectly normal foal would not have enough of a weakness there

125

to allow the "creation" of a hernia, it could also be argued that the problem was actually an acquired condition of the umbilical cord itself, causing it to be abnormally thickened and tough, making it resistant to normal separation.

Diagnostically, determining whether an umbilical hernia is congenital or acquired is difficult and ticklish, since the ramifications of a congenital condition can be damaging to the reputations of the foal's parents. Frankly, most umbilical hernias are congenital, and most congenital hernias don't become obvious until the foal is a day or two old. Regardless of their cause, most get smaller over time, but some stay the same or get larger, requiring surgical repair in order to prevent problems with entrapment of bowel.

In any case, it seems that the informed and responsible thing to do is to attempt to prevent damage to the abdominal wall of the foal as the umbilical cord breaks. This is easily accomplished by gently placing your hand against the foal's abdomen, palm side to tummy, at the point where the umbilical cord is attached to the foal. Allow the umbilical cord to run between two fingers, but do not squeeze it with those fingers, since this would interfere with the flow of blood through the cord. By applying just enough gentle pressure against the foal's abdomen with the palm of your hand to counteract the tension being exerted on it by the stretched umbilical cord, you can protect the abdomen while allowing the cord to begin its slow, gradual tearing. If the umbilical cord has no tension on it at this particular moment, leave your hand in its supportive position, but apply no support until it is needed. The foal will become accustomed to the presence of your hand and will not be disturbed by it.

When the mare prepares to stand up, remember that this will pull the umbilical cord taut and may actually cause the foal to be pulled along the ground a bit from the strength of the tug. Be prepared to support the foal's abdomen against the tension, and as soon as the cord breaks, grasp the stump that remains attached to the foal and squirt it generously with your iodine solution, giving it a good soaking. Get your head in there and watch the tip of the stump for bleeding. Do not rely on looking at the foal's legs for bloodstains to tell you if the stump is bleeding, since they may have some blood spilled on them by the *other* end of the umbilical stump when it breaks. It is expected that some of the blood that accumulated in the upper portion of the umbilical cord, closer to the mare, will spill out when the cord breaks.

The foal's stump may ooze a little bit for less than a minute, which is acceptable, but if the flow of blood is more purposeful than just an ooze, you will have to tie the stump off with your short piece of clean cotton string. Foals invariably become extremely active just at the moment when you need to do something rather delicate such as tie a hemorrhaging umbilical stump, so prepare to be frustrated

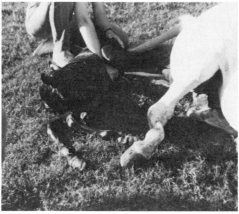

FIGURE 4.57
The umbilical cord must have tension on it in order for it to break. In some cases excessive and/or prolonged tension on the umbilical cord "pulls a hernia" in the foal's abdominal wall. Gentle palm pressure against the foal's abdomen can protect it from damage until the cord breaks.

as the foal confounds your efforts to get it tied off quickly. If possible, get your assistant to hold the foal's upper rear leg away from your vulnerable face while you loop your string around the midsection of the umbilical stump. Without pulling on the foal's abdomen, tie the string snugly and pull the knot tight. After you have assured yourself that the string is tied securely and there is no more blood leakage, give the entire stump another good soaking with your iodine solution. **This iodine soaking should be repeated at least twice more within the next couple of hours** whether or not the stump was tied.

Don't be surprised the next time you treat the stump with iodine to find that the string is gone—in most cases it tends to fall off by itself within a very short period of time when the portion of the stump distal to the string falls

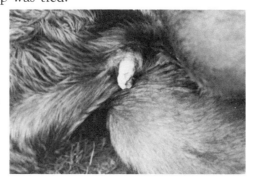

FIGURE 4.58
The umbilical cord stump should be tied off only if it is bleeding, and only if the bleeding persists for more than a moment. This stump is perfectly normal and needs no tie (ligature).

off. This is almost never accompanied by a resumption of bleeding, since it only seems necessary to pinch the umbilical stump for a couple of minutes to get the ruptured end to clot and seal

127

over permanently. If, however, the string manages to stay on the stump for more than a few hours, it should be removed, since it is porous and may permit bacteria to travel, wicklike, up the string to the umbilical cord. This is a good job for your veterinarian if you are unsteady with knots or scissors. Once again, treat the stump with your iodine solution after removing the string.

The assertion that the umbilical cord should remain intact for 10 minutes after the foal is born is based on the belief that the foal is still receiving valuable blood through the umbilical cord even after it has begun to air-breathe independently of its mother. It is possible to feel the cord pulsate during the first few minutes after the foal has emerged, but it is not certain whether the pulsations indicate that blood is actually flowing through the cord into the foal, whether the pulsations are merely an "echo" or backwash of the blood that is now being blocked at the foal's umbilicus, or whether the pulsations are only muscular in origin.

It has long been believed that if the umbilical cord ruptures before the pulsations stop, the foal will be "robbed" of up to a pint of blood, potentially contributing to weakness and poor disease resistance during those crucial first days of life. However, recent research has tested the red blood cell count of foals whose umbilical cords were purposely cut at various times, ranging from immediately after birth to more than 10 minutes after birth, and there was no significant difference in the blood counts of the various treatment groups. With what is already known about the change in the source of oxygen supply in the foal immediately after birth, the umbilical cord is unlikely to be a significant source of blood for the newborn foal. It is more likely that a certain amount of blood is routinely "trapped" in the length of umbilical cord between the mare and the foal when the foal is born, and the trapped blood is simply expected to be wasted. When the umbilical cord ruptures "early," this trapped blood has not yet had time to clot, and it spills onto the mare's hocks and the foal's torso and all over the ground and looks like a *lot* of blood. If the umbilical cord remains intact for 5 minutes or so before rupturing, a portion of the trapped blood becomes clotted, and very little is spilled out when the cord finally ruptures.

Having said all that, however, it is still advised that the mare and foal be encouraged to lie quietly and protect the umbilical cord for ten minutes or so after birth, since both have been through a significant physical ordeal and can use the time to recuperate and make, in the foal's case, some important adjustments. Additionally, the "dotted line" on the umbilical cord where separation usually takes place seems to mature as the minutes pass, becoming more easily separated with each passing minute. This has the advantage of allowing the cord to rupture before excessive tension is placed on the foal's tender abdomen, lessening the chance of creating an acquired umbilical hernia. Furthermore, and most importantly, the umbilical stump on the foal's abdomen is much more likely to hemorrhage if rupture occurs too soon after birth, causing the rapid and alarming loss of blood that already "belonged" to the foal and necessitating that you tie the stump off before too much blood is lost. And finally, consider that when human interference is kept at a minimum, most mares choose to stay down and rest, sometimes remaining relaxed and quiet for thirty minutes or more before returning to their vigilant duties as nervous guardians against real or imagined enemies. It simply seems unfair to deprive them of this peaceful time when the only requirement is that we humans restrict our activity and noise level to a sensitive minimum.

Foal Restraint

It is important that your first encounters with the newborn be as relaxed and free of trauma as possible. In general it is best to approach very young foals with your body bent slightly over in a "hunched" posture to minimize your intimidating human height. As a rule, one arm cradled gently around the front of the foal's chest to keep him from going forward is the most effective restraint, since the goal should be to coax the foal into cooperating rather than to force him to your will and alarm him. If more restraint is needed, the next level is to add your other arm over the withers, placing the palm of your open hand against the far shoulder to press the foal toward you in a gentle embrace. Young foals tend to toss their heads about quickly and somewhat explosively, so keep your head pressed against the foal to avoid being "conked." If long-term restraint is needed, such as for transporting the foal to another pasture, it is sometimes effective to apply a full-size horse halter to the foal's torso. The chin-strap portion of the halter, which is situated along the foal's withers, can be used as a handle for guiding the foal. This is surprisingly well tolerated by most neonatal foals.

For injections and other painful procedures that usually require forceful restraint, leave the forward arm around the front of the foal's chest and place your other arm around the foal's hindquarters just below the buttocks. With your arms in this position, it is possible (and sometimes necessary) to actually lift the foal up off the ground and hold him in your arms.

In some cases, rather than placing the arm around the hindquarters, it is more effective to hold the tail in the upright position close to its base. The intent is not to use the tail as a "handle," since damage to its vertebrae and nerve supply would be a sorry side effect of such mishandling. In order to minimize the risk of such damage, the tail should be held only at its base, as close to its attachment to the foal's body as possible. However, holding the tail in the upright position is, in some cases, an effective means of "taking the foal out of gear," much the same way that a twitch applied to the upper lip of an adult horse seems to place him into a light hypnotic state.

If you are qualified to give intramuscular injections, or if your veterinarian is present at the birthing, **it is a good idea to give the foal's tetanus antitoxin injection as early as possible**, since the *Clostridium tetani* bacteria that cause tetanus are ubiquitous in horse facilities and since the fresh umbilical stump is a perfect avenue for the bacteria to enter the newborn foal's bloodstream. Opponents of this procedure argue that the foal will receive antibodies from the mare's first milk (colostrum) to protect against tetanus, but the many factors that may intervene to delay or prevent the foal from receiving this protection from the milk are sufficient to encourage using the injection as an additional safeguard. Furthermore, nobody who has seen a foal with tetanus would ever argue against giving this inexpensive, relatively safe injection. The disease itself is horrible, extremely expensive to treat, usually fatal and ridiculously easy to prevent.

Since the newborn foal is disoriented and relatively insensitive to painful stimuli during its first few minutes of life, it is easy and stress-free to give the tetanus antitoxin injection right away, as soon as the foal has emerged from the mare and is safely breathing on his own. If it is possible to perform this simple task without disturbing the mare during her important rest phase, then it is advised to go ahead and do it. This should only be done by persons with experience in the proper technique of giving intramuscular injections, since it is always important to avoid accidental injection into an artery or vein, damage to nerve fibers, and/or infection at the injection site. The best site for the qualified operator to give the newborn foal its tetanus antitoxin injection is a clean spot on the muscles of the back of the thigh (semimembranosis/semitendinosis muscles), taking special care to pinch the muscles away from the sciatic nerve and insert the needle at an angle from front (anterior) to back (posterior) to ensure that the nerve is not penetrated. As always when giving intramuscular injections, the needle should be inserted separately, detached from the syringe, checked for backflow of blood, then attached to the syringe and checked once again for blood by pulling back on the plunger before administering the injection (see Figures 4.59 through 4.61).

ENEMA

At this point, you have taken care of two of the three basic tasks in newborn foal care that must be attended to during the immediate post-birthing period:

1. Examining and treating the umbilical stump.
2. Administering the tetanus antitoxin injection (to be done only by a qualified person).
3. The third task is to administer an enema, since the foal's colon contains fecal matter (meconium), which is relatively dry, hard and a potential source of impaction colic.

Most mammals, regardless of species, respond to a natural reflex which stimulates the colon to evacuate when food enters the stomach, thus creating the urge to defecate after taking a meal. The same is true of newborn foals, and the first milk meal suckled from their mothers is usually followed by their first bowel movement. This process is called the gastrocolonic reflex, and it is the basis of many training techniques striving to toilet-train human babies and housetrain puppies, showing them the proper place to defecate immediately after feeding. Nevertheless, there

FIGURE 4.59 A,B
With the rear muscles of the thigh pinched in this manner, important structures such as the sciatic nerve are pushed forward, away from the needle. The needle is aimed toward the back as an added safety measure.

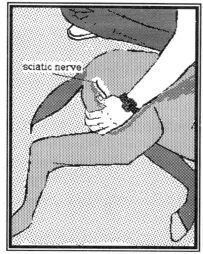

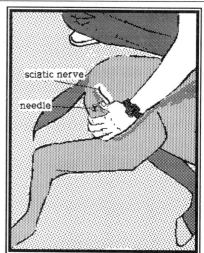

FIGURE 4.60 A,B
After attaching the syringe to the needle, pull back on the plunger to make sure the needle has not penetrated an artery or vein. If blood enters the syringe, remove the needle and start over with a fresh one.

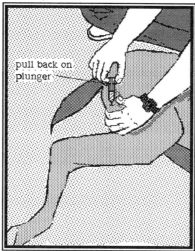

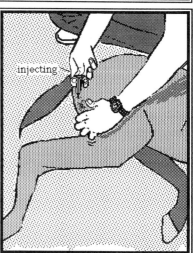

are numerous factors that may interfere with the timely evacuation of the newborn's colon, the consequences of which are serious and potentially life-threatening. The administration of an enema is simple, safe and inexpensive insurance against impaction colic, and since an enema will produce results within a reasonably short period of time, it is easy to evaluate the effectiveness of your treatment and decide whether a second treatment is warranted. If results are not satisfactory within two treatments and an hour's time, veterinary intervention should be sought to determine if a problem already exists. Without the advantage of early detection provided by the enema, a problem may go undetected until the impaction colic is advanced enough

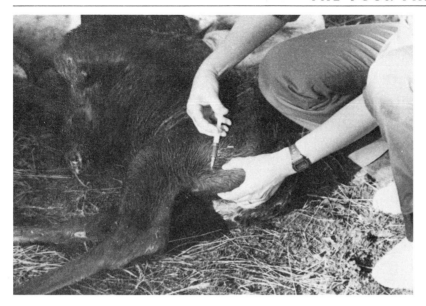

FIGURE 4.61
The injection should be given only after all safety measures have been taken. Don't let the objections of the mare or foal convince you to be hasty.

to produce painful colic symptoms in the foal. The routine administration of an enema to a newborn foal forces the foaling attendant to consider and watch for the foal's first manure. It also forces the attendant to check for atresia ani, a birth defect in which the foal is born with an anus that is sealed closed.

The most commonly used enema in newborn foals is the adult human Fleet enema, a phosphate-based liquid in a soft, pliable plastic container with a prelubricated, blunt tip for insertion directly into the rectum. The convenience, effectiveness and low cost of this product make it perfect for application in treating newborn foals. The smaller quantity in the child-size Fleet is usually insufficient for the newborn foal, so it is better to keep a few of the adult-size Fleets on hand during foaling season.

Although the administration of an enema is considered to be part of the "immediate postfoaling" regimen, **wait until the foal is standing on his own, usually within an hour of birth, before giving the enema.** The reason for postponing the enema until this time relates to the straining that most foals must do in order to push out their first manure. Meconium is tacky and hard, and the newborn foal's "pucker string" (anus) is usually rather tight at first. As a result, the first bowel movement is often associated with substantial effort, even when given the assistance of an enema. The increased pushing can cause the umbilical stump to begin bleeding if the foal's efforts start before the

133

stump is solidly clotted and sealed. This is usually not a significant problem, but it is easy to avoid the problem completely by simply waiting until the foal is standing to administer the enema. Very little restraint is needed for this procedure.

If it is very cold outside, prewarm the enema by immersing the sealed Fleet in a container of lukewarm water for 15 minutes or so before administering it. The nozzle of the Fleet enema is sealed with a pale green plastic cap, which must be removed to expose the open nozzle before administering the enema. To give the enema, have your assistant corral the frolicking foal gently in his or her arms. You can then approach quietly from behind your assistant and gently lift the foal's tail with one hand just enough to expose his anus. With the other hand, slowly insert the nozzle of the Fleet into the anus (be sure it isn't going into the vagina, if it's a filly!), relax the hold on the foal's tail and squeeze the enema into the rectum with a single firm squeeze. (In many instances, if you have to change your grip on the enema bottle for a second squeeze, the foal will begin to push the liquid out before it has had a chance to work and soften the hard little

FIGURE 4.62
Use only as much restraint as is needed to safely accomplish the task at hand. It may only be necessary to "corral" the foal loosely with one arm, or a gentle but firm embrace may be warranted.

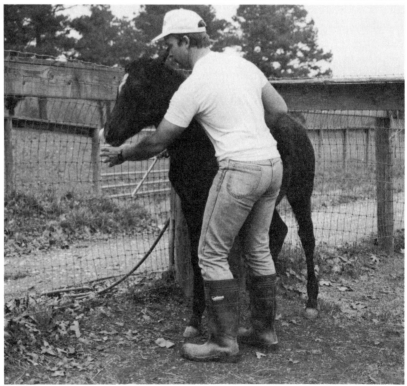

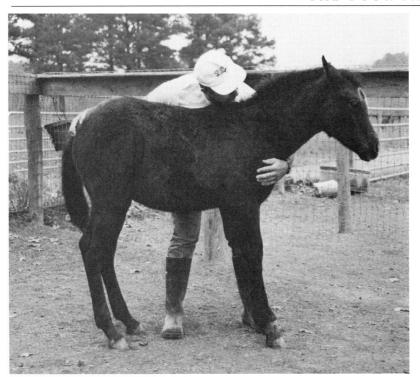

FIGURE 4.63
The "bear hug" hold is more effective for certain procedures and, if necessary, the foal can actually be lifted off the ground and carried in this position. Note that the handler's head is close to the foal in order to avoid being "conked" by the foal's head.

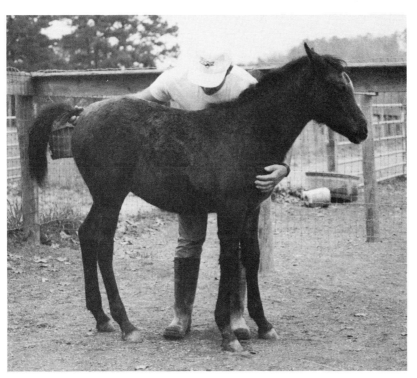

FIGURE 4.64
For procedures that are likely to be resented, such as intravenous injections or blood tests, the proper tail hold can be an effective and safe means of restraint.

135

Special note: For obvious impactions that do not apparently respond to Fleet or soapy water enemas, a somewhat expensive but very effective alternative is an enema made with acetylcysteine (an agent that is also used to break up mucus in the lungs of patients with pneumonia). A solution of 1 heaping tablespoon of acetylcysteine powder, mixed with 24 ounces of water, and buffered with 1.5 level tablespoons of baking soda, is administered deep into the rectum using a soft 30-French Foley catheter. This treatment is also used in human babies with meconium impactions, and it has been very effective. The powder may be difficult to obtain—best to get some well in advance. Chemical supply houses and pharmacies would be a good place to start looking.

manure balls.) Release the tail, remove the nozzle from the foal's anus and walk away. Most professional horse trainers agree that your assistant should wait a moment before releasing the foal in order to gradually acclimate the foal to gentle restraint and to show him that restraint is not necessarily associated with having some procedure "done to him."

The best, most effective enemas are enemas that remain in the rectum for a little while to soften the manure before the evacuation begins. The amount of meconium passed by newborn foals tends to exceed most expectations, and it is not unusual for a single enema to induce the passage of three or four or five piles over an hour's time that, when combined, would nearly fill a half-gallon milk carton. This tends to vary with geographical location for some reason—the total volume of meconium seems to be higher in some regions of the country than in others.

If the foal is having difficulty passing the meconium, he will generally demonstrate discomfort by swishing his tail excessively, posturing to defecate and straining, sometimes with an audible groan, with little or no results. Occasionally the administration of the enema is followed with absolutely no response at all—no discomfort, no effort and no meconium. In either case, it is perfectly reasonable to give another enema, but **do not give a second Fleet enema unless the bulk of the first Fleet has been pushed out.** This is because the chemical agent in Fleet-type enemas, which is ordinarily quite safe, can become toxic if excessive amounts of it are absorbed into the circulation. If the first Fleet remains in the rectum and additional doses are given with no results, it is possible that too much of the phosphates will be absorbed and approach toxic levels. Therefore, any enemas given after the first Fleet should be warm soapy water enemas, which are simple to prepare. Using the flexible plastic bottle from the Fleet enema already given, place a drop or two of Ivory liquid soap (not detergent) into the bottle, fill with lukewarm water, shake it up until well mixed and administer in the same manner as the first enema.

In most cases, the second enema produces the desired results. However, if the foal is still visibly uncomfortable and has not produced sufficient meconium (at least a pint), veterinary attention is definitely warranted and should already have been requested. If, on the other hand, little meconium has been passed but the foal seems perfectly comfortable, it is possible that the meconium is higher up in the foal's intestines, slightly out of reach of the enema's effects. In this case, the situation is usually resolved with the aid of the gastrocolonic reflex, and as soon as the foal takes his first sizable milk meal, the passage of a large batch of meconium should not be far behind.

The gastrocolonic reflex must compete with another natural response, which may cause a short delay in the passage of the foal's meconium. Most newborn foals will lie down and sleep deeply for 20 or 30 minutes after a nice long milk meal. In some cases, particularly when the mare's milk is running profusely, the need for a nap will hit the foal "like a ton of bricks" and he will appear suddenly overcome with sleepiness. In most cases after a deep sleep, the foal will rise and immediately pass a large volume of meconium.

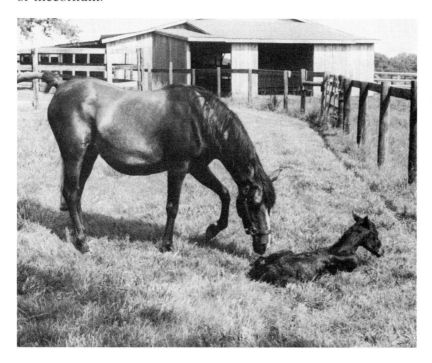

FIGURE 4.65
Almost immediately after finally getting a satisfying milk meal, many foals will appear suddenly overcome with sleepiness.

HEALTH SAFEGUARDS FOR THE FOAL

Some of the larger breeding farms have instituted the policy of giving every newborn foal an injection of antibiotics (usually penicillin) and/or vitamins (usually B-complex vitamins) routinely after birth. The reasoning behind this policy is likely to be a well-meaning but misinformed attempt at preventing foal ill-nesses. Research has shown that the routine administration of antibiotics and vitamins to newborn foals is *not* associated with less disease. In fact, **there is a statistically significant increase in the number of foals getting diarrhea within groups getting the antibiotic injections routinely at birth.** Furthermore, allergic-type sensitivity to penicillin and other agents is not uncommon in horses, and the odds of encountering a sensitive individual increase with each injection given. The most severe kind of allergic reaction, called an anaphylactic reaction, is very dra-matic and usually fatal.

One practice that has been shown to decrease the inci-dence of foal diarrhea is washing (and rinsing) the mare's udder before the foal's first suckle. This is especially important during the fly season, since the mare's udder is often sweaty and a favorite target for flies, which have already soiled their little feet on filth and manure piles. Well-meaning caretakers may have used fly repellants and/or insecticides on the mare's underside to provide some relief from the blood-sucking marauders, and these agents should *definitely* be washed off before the newborn foal's lips get anywhere near the udder. By the same token, most foals spend a lot of time mouthing their mothers in areas that are nowhere near the udder until they finally find the "cafeteria." For this reason, some serious thought should be given to getting the chemicals off the mare's entire body before the foal is born.

Better yet, try to institute fly control by using some method other than chemical warfare. The most effective fly control has always been fastidiousness, and especially in the case of pregnant mares, keeping the barn clean has many benefits beyond fly con-trol. The use of fly predators, otherwise harmless insects that feed on fly larvae, has also been very successful in controlling fly populations in the stable, to the extent that even very filthy barns full of manure have surprisingly low fly populations when adequately "seeded" with fly predators. Disposal of manure in composting piles well away from the barn is essential.

Regardless of the level of your experience and expertise in foal-ing attendance, the feelings of relief and accomplishment are understandably palpable at this point. However, this is not the time for champagne, bright lights, flash cameras, back slapping and telephoned invitations to friends to come see the new foal. There are still some very important steps that must take place without excessive interference and without a break in your concentration. So leave the lights dimmed, keep the audience at bay, keep the noise down and enter Stage III.

Section 4.7
Fourth Phase—Stage III, Passing the Placenta

Try to imagine what the inside of the mare's uterus looks like now. The dark red, villous surface of the allantois-chorion is still closely attached to the lining of the uterus, as though the pregnancy were still intact, but the portion of the sac closest to the mare's cervix now has a large gaping hole through which the foal escaped. The inner surface of the allantois-chorion, which is the smooth, lavender-colored, rubber-like surface, surrounds a space that once housed the foal in his flimsy amnion but that is now vacuous and sloshy, containing a gallon or more of retained allantoic fluid. Most of the amnion came out with the foal, but

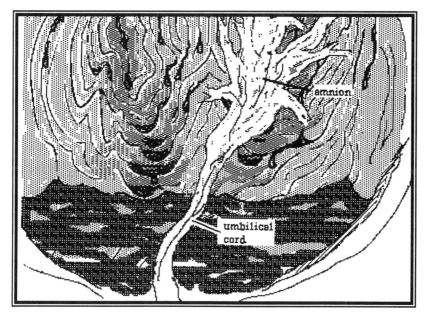

FIGURE 4.66
The inside of the mare's uterus is now very different than it was a moment ago. The allantois-chorion is still attached, but before long it will start to loosen as the uterus begins to contract, turning itself inside out as it pushes the heavy membranes out.

139

the umbilical cord, which is now hanging out of the mare's vulva, is still attached at its other end to one horn of the allantois-chorion. This is the only "handle" that we have on the allantois-chorion (now called the "afterbirth"), and it is not strong enough to endure significant tension. In other words, it would not be possible to pull the afterbirth out by pulling on the umbilical cord, because the afterbirth is still attached, like Velcro, to the uterus, and because the umbilical cord would break if you pulled on it very hard. Furthermore, if the umbilical cord were strong enough to permit much tension, chances are that in addition to pulling out the afterbirth, you would also pull out the uterus, since the uterus must first release the afterbirth from its Velcro-like attachments before the afterbirth can be expelled.

In actuality, the afterbirth comes out because the uterus pushes it out. No manner of pulling will retrieve it until the uterus is ready and able to push, because the Velcro-like attachment of the afterbirth to the uterus is very strong, and because the afterbirth must come uphill, from the abdomen to the pelvic canal, before it can come out. Nevertheless, the weight of the umbilical cord and amnion hanging out of the mare's vulva is very important in getting the afterbirth out. This is *not* because

FIGURE 4.67 A,B
Normally, placental detachment from the uterus involves some resistance but not enough to result in tearing. If the detachment of the placenta is delayed for any reason, the inflammatory processes taking place in the uterus cause uterine swelling, uterine crypt tightening and, in turn, swelling of the placental villi, which are now being "pinched" in their crypts. Thus detachment becomes more and more difficult.

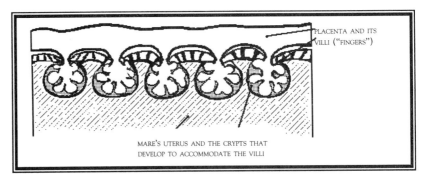

PLACENTA AND ITS VILLI ("FINGERS")

MARE'S UTERUS AND THE CRYPTS THAT
DEVELOP TO ACCOMMODATE THE VILLI

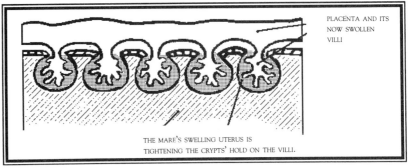

PLACENTA AND ITS
NOW SWOLLEN
VILLI

THE MARE'S SWELLING UTERUS IS
TIGHTENING THE CRYPTS' HOLD ON THE VILLI.

140

the weight pulls the afterbirth out, but rather because it makes the mare uncomfortable and tends to remind her that the afterbirth must be passed. Even though uterine contractions, which are involuntary, are instrumental in expelling the afterbirth, a certain amount of willful cooperation on the part of the mare is also necessary. If the mare is distracted in any way, whether by worrying over her newborn foal, listening to faraway sounds or concerning herself with the human activity around her, she can postpone her work on the afterbirth. This has dire consequences, because the longer the afterbirth remains in the uterus, the more inflamed the uterus becomes. Inflammation is always associated with a certain degree of swelling, and when the uterus begins to swell because of inflammation, the Velcro-like attachment of the afterbirth to the uterus will begin to get very tight (see Figure 4.70 a and b). Therefore, the longer the afterbirth remains attached to the uterus, the more difficult it will be to "undo" the attachment.

It has been demonstrated that the afterbirth also can act as a "wick" for bacteria and other contaminants, so that the potential for uterine contamination slowly creeps up the afterbirth toward the uterus as long as the afterbirth remains attached. This is primarily the result of capillary action, and the process seems to be accelerated when the ambient temperature is higher. The potential for a resultant uterine infection is higher in warm weather, since bacteria multiply faster in higher temperatures. Therefore, the longer the afterbirth remains attached to the uterus, the higher the risk that the uterus will become infected.

Therefore, do everything possible to encourage the mare to work on passing the afterbirth. Since the afterbirth must come uphill before it can come out, passage generally happens much faster if the mare is lying down, because gravity is no longer working against her. However, it is an established fact that horses are, in general, reluctant to lie down because of heightened vulnerability. This is especially true of mares with newborn foals, and yet it is even more important for their futures as broodmares to lie down as soon as possible and get that afterbirth out. For this reason, it is essential that the noise and activity and other distractions be maintained at an absolute minimum during Stage III.

It is always advisable to wear plastic gloves when handling

141

any of the birth tissues, including the afterbirth, since on occasion such tissues may harbor infectious organisms that can threaten human health as well as the health of other animals you may handle. Undulant fever (brucellosis) is an example of a disease that can be transmitted from an animal species to humans (a zoonotic disease), and although it is less common in horses than in other domestic animals, it is much better to avoid the possibility of contact with it than to face a future of uncertain health from this persistent, resistant disease.

If the umbilical cord and amnion that are hanging out of the mare's vulva are allowed to drag on the ground, the mare may step on them and slip, endangering the safety of the foal, and she may break part of them off. In order to prevent any banana-peel falls, and in order to preserve as much as possible of the weight of these membranes, **you should tie up the afterbirth with your long piece of clean cotton string.** Some people tie the membranes into a big "bunch" and then tie the bunch to the mare's tail, but this obviously would not allow the full weight of the membranes to pull on the mare's birth canal and would not serve to stimulate afterbirth passage. With your trusted attendant at the mare's head, tie the string around the end of the membranes, then lift the tied portion up off the ground and tie it up high on the membranes as they emerge from the vulva. If this leaves a loop that is longer than hock level on the mare, lift the end up and incorporate it in another knot at the vulva. If any of the "purple part" of the afterbirth is protruding from the vulva, try your best to incorporate this in your knot, since this is the portion of the afterbirth that must be passed first in order for the rest to follow. If the purple part is included in your knot, the time required for afterbirth passage will be much shorter.

If it is warm outside, and if flies are present, you may want to enclose the tied-up membranes in a long plastic glove or bag that is secured with another string. Some mares are nervous about plastic rustling around their hindquarters, but if your mare tolerates this well, there will be much less blood and serum soiling her tail and hindquarters and much less bait for marauding flies.

As a general rule, the afterbirth should be completely out within two hours of the foal's birth for the process to be considered perfectly normal, and it is preferable that it be out within

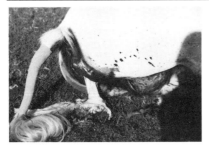 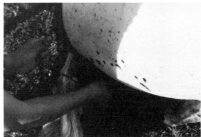

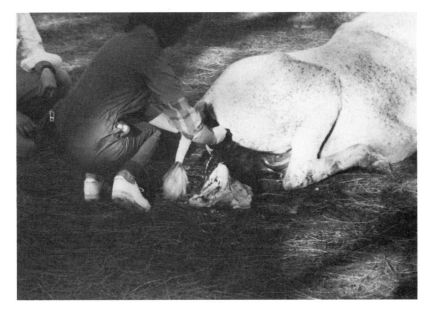

FIGURE 4.68 A,B.& C
Tie the long cotton string to the end of the amnionic portion of the afterbirth, then bring that end up and tie it close to the mare's vulva. If it's still too long, bring the bottom of the looped amnion up to the string and tie it into the knot.

If the "purple part" (the allantois-chorion) is (or becomes) visible at the lips of the vulva, try to incorporate it into the knot as well.

Each of these steps will require a separate knot but using the same string if it's long enough.

one hour. The warmer the weather, the more important it is that the length of Stage III be shorter so that the risk of uterine infection from ascending contaminants is minimized. Nevertheless, **the temptation to pull on the portion of the afterbirth that is already exposed should be resisted**, since this is almost never productive and increases the risk that damage will be done to the mare's uterus. **The most effective way to speed up the process of passing the afterbirth is to make it as easy as possible for the mare to lie down,** since her horizontal position makes it easier for the purple (allantois-chorion) portion of the afterbirth, which has become detached from the uterus, to slip out and provide additional weight. It is not uncommon for a mare to stand spraddle-legged and strain mightily in an effort to pass the afterbirth, and make absolutely no visible progress, but when she lies down even for a brief time, there will be considerably more

143

afterbirth hanging out when she stands up again. Progress is almost assured with every time the mare goes down.

The frustration of Stage III attendance is palpable when the mare begins to turn around and around, preparing to lie down, starts to lower herself to the ground, then is suddenly distracted by some tiny little annoyance—a distant dog barking, a horse

FIGURE 4.69
With gravity working to keep the afterbirth in the uterus, the mare's uterine contractions are much less effective at expelling the afterbirth if she is standing. Once she lies down, any portion of the allantois-chorion that already detached from the uterus is better able to spill out, and when the mare stands up again, this new portion will contribute its considerable weight to coaxing the remaining membranes out as soon as they detach.

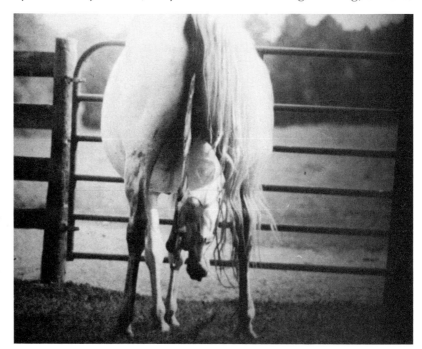

neighing, a telephone ringing, the foal disturbing her, somebody whispering just a little too loudly—and she decides not to lie down just yet. This scenario repeats itself over and over during the course of Stage III, and with each foaling experience you will find yourself becoming more and more sensitive to all the little interferences that exist in your environment. It is definitely advisable, therefore, to keep the area as quiet, dimly lit and interference-free as possible.

For this reason, refrain from giving the mare her after-foaling bran mash until the afterbirth is out. Try to discourage the foal from nursing until then, since it will probably take him several tries before he gets enough milk to satisfy himself, and his repeated efforts will only distract the mare from passing the afterbirth. (There is scientific evidence to suggest that milk let-down is encouraged after the afterbirth has detached from the uterus, so the foal's nursing efforts are much more likely to be rewarded generously if he will wait until the afterbirth is out.) Furthermore, most mares are preoccupied with their discomfort and moderately less receptive to the foal's nursing attempts until after the afterbirth is out. If the foal is precocious and persistent and/or if the afterbirth is very slow to come out, the foal may become a significant interference to the mare's concentration, prolonging Stage III unnecessarily, and it may be helpful to milk 4 or 6 ounces of the mare's colostrum into a baby bottle and give it to the foal so that he will lie down and take a half-hour nap. For help in accomplishing this, see Section 5.1.

There are two reasons for a delay in passing the afterbirth. The most common reason is apprehension/anxiety/preoccupation on the part of the mare, preventing her from lying down or posturing to push out the already loosened portion of the placenta. Ordinarily, the added weight of this part of the placenta helps in the systematic detachment of the remaining part and also helps to stimulate the uterus to continue detaching and pushing. As discussed earlier in this section, if the detachment is delayed for too long, even when there is no underlying disease process, the tissues involved in the union become swollen and more tightly attached to each other, making separation more difficult to accomplish. The most obvious solution to this problem is to prevent it by providing the mare with the kind of environment that encourages her to focus on her tasks and minimizes the distractions and feelings of vulnerability associated with lying down. If more than an hour passes and no progress is made despite obvious effort on the mare's part, the possibility exists that the second reason prevails: a portion of the afterbirth is actually "stuck" to the uterus because of some previous inflammation or infection, and veterinary intervention will be needed to separate it.

As soon as the afterbirth falls to the ground, remove it from the nursery area so that neither the foal nor the mare will step on it. (However, be prepared to return it to the stall if the mare's behavior toward the foal is overly suspicious or aggressive. For more information, see Section 5.3.) Although some mares will show an interest in chewing on the afterbirth, it is not a sustained interest, and there seems to be no benefit in allowing the mare to indulge. Postparturient constipation has been known to

145

occur in many species, partly because of the dehydrating effect of heavy lactation (milking). Eating the afterbirth may have a laxative effect, but since horses are so sensitive to abdominal discomfort, it seems more prudent to remove the afterbirth and offer the mare a nice, fresh, juicy-sloppy warm bran mash instead.

The afterbirth should be examined to ascertain whether it contains any areas of infection and/or if any pieces are missing, such as a small patch that may have become too tightly adhered to the uterus, tearing away from the rest of the afterbirth and remaining adhered to the lining of the uterus. In this instance, the mare will require veterinary treatment in order to prevent uterine infection from the presence of the rotting piece of retained afterbirth. Examining the afterbirth will also give indication of other abnormalities such as existing infection of the placental tissues or uterus. Nonveterinary attendants should examine the afterbirth as well, since its appearance will change as it begins to dry and decompose and there may be a delay before the veterinarian has a chance to look at it. Furthermore, laying out the afterbirth in its original position can be very educational and can reinforce what is already known about the appearance and functional relationship among uterus, placenta and fetus.

Lay the afterbirth out on a clean, level surface in its original T-shape, with the torn cervical star facing you and the horns spreading out away from you to the left and right. Unless you inverted it, the allantois-chorion part of the afterbirth will be inside out, the way it was passed, the purple part on the outside. While still inside the mare, remember, the purple part was on the inside, facing the foal, and the deep red, roughened part was on the outside, attached like Velcro to the lining of the uterus. The flimsy whitish part, the amnion, was a separate sac inside the

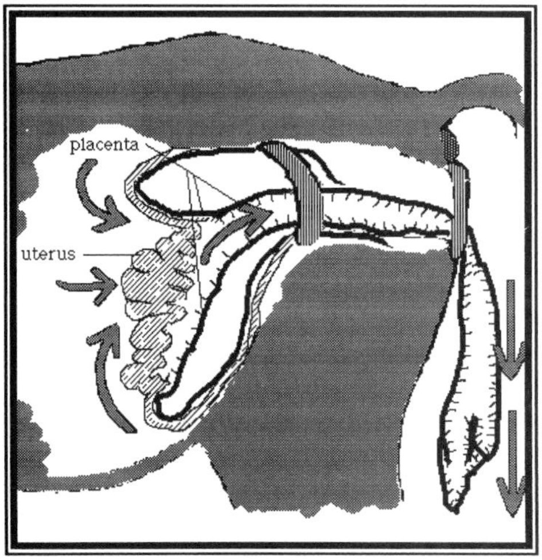

FIGURE 4.70
As more and more of the afterbirth detaches and slips out of the vagina, its weight pulls on the remaining portion that is still attached. If a section is attached too tightly, the weight may pull on it enough to pull the uterus out. Any attempts to encourage passage of the afterbirth should be done with this possibility foremost in mind.

placenta

uterus

146

allantois-chorion, and you should find that it has two ends—the broken-off umbilical end, which had been attached to the foal's abdomen, and the end of origin, which emanates like roots from the central portion of the "ceiling" of the allantois-chorion. More specifically, it originates from the purple surface, slightly to one side of the center of the "crotch" or bifurcation in the T-shape. This corresponds to the site where the early pregnancy implanted in the uterus during its second or third week of life.

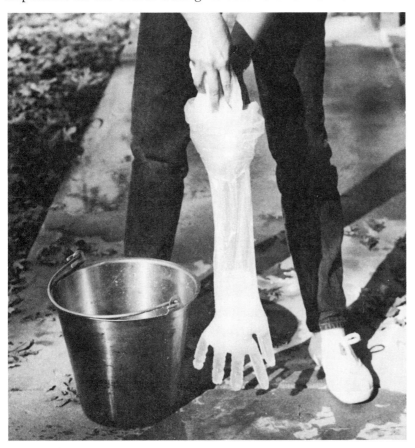

FIGURE 4.71
The typical waterbag weight is no more than two pounds, made conveniently with a plastic disposable rectal glove filled to the wrist with water or water-soaked cotton, then tied to the exposed amnionic portion of the afterbirth.

   Intervention to resolve a case of retained fetal membranes (RFM) in the mare differs from the same situation in the cow. In the cow, the RFM may persist for a day or longer, becoming quite rotted and fetid, and it usually can be removed manually by carefully and laboriously unbuttoning the adhered membrane from the uterus and removing it, intact or piece by piece. Most cows will not exhibit signs of general illness despite all the rot and gore taking place in the uterus. Mares, however, will become

147

quite ill and will generally exhibit serious signs of toxicity within 12 to 24 hours when even a small piece of placenta is retained. Manual removal is usually not possible, nor is it recommended, and intervention is aimed at (1) encouraging the stubborn attachment to separate, and/or (2) administering preventive medicine to keep the mare from getting sick while waiting for the membrane to be expelled after exhaustive efforts to retrieve it have failed.

The most rational approach to encourage detachment when the retained placenta is still in one piece involves gradually increasing the intervention while standing by at all times to observe the results before trying the next step. There is always the possibility that a portion of the placenta is irretrievably adhered to the uterus, and this carries with it the probability that when the rest of the placenta finally detaches and slips out, its weight will pull on the adhered portion and pull the uterus out. This requires quick action and a clear head, manually detaching the small adhered portion and pushing the uterus back in before a true uterine prolapse occurs (see pages 151–159). In most cases, however, the stubbornly attached areas will finally, reluctantly let go in response to the veterinarian's intervention. Most veterinarians will employ these procedures to encourage passage of the afterbirth:

Special note: Passage of the afterbirth is associated with natural oxytocin release by the mare's own pituitary gland. This also causes milk letdown. By the same token, a viable "treatment" for retained placenta is to milk four to six ounces of colostrum into a bottle for the foal, since the oxytocin release associated with milk letdown may be just the ticket for stimulating the uterus to push the retained placenta out.

1. If the mare seems distracted and has made little effort in passing the afterbirth, the judicious use of a "waterbag" weight on the exposed amnionic portion of the afterbirth is often sufficient stimulus to encourage a shift in the mare's focus, augmenting the uterine contractions with willful posturing, abdominal press and recumbency. The function of the weight is *not* to pull the afterbirth out—this would never succeed. In fact, **if too much weight is applied, the afterbirth will tear, the exposed portion will fall to the ground, and the remaining portion will slip back into the uterus and evade further attempts at retrieval**. The veterinarian, exercising judgment in deciding how much weight to add, usually pours sufficient water (or water-soaked cotton) into a plastic disposable rectal sleeve to fill it just past the base of the thumb. The sleeve is then tied in a knot, placed inside a second sleeve to prevent leakage, then tied onto the exposed amnionic portion of the afterbirth. This method is rational only

if the allantois-chorion ("purple part") is not visible externally; i.e., **the waterbag approach should never be used if the purple part has begun to protrude from the vagina**. This is because the uterus is definitely contracting in order to expose the purple, which means that it has begun to bunch itself up and push itself toward the mare's rear. Any added weight at this point may apply too much tension on the uterus and pull it too close to the outside, encouraging a prolapse. The veterinarian should stand by with scissors to cut the waterbag open and drain out the water if the added weight seems to be having an unexpected or unwanted effect. Additionally, some mares are made uneasy by the plastic waterbag rustling and bumping their hocks, and the overall effect may actually contribute to their distraction rather than to help them focus on passing the afterbirth.

2. Directly pulling on the afterbirth is prohibited, since it does nothing to encourage detachment of the placenta from the uterus, yet it does much to encourage the uterus to prolapse. In selected cases, however, the veterinarian may choose to apply twisting (torsion) to the exposed purple portion of the afterbirth, since this can encourage detachment without risking prolapse. If the afterbirth is diseased or infected, however, it may be fragile and easily torn (friable) and the operator must be careful not to twist too vigorously and cause tearing. When warranted, the twisting is done slowly and methodically, first rolling the exposed membranes all the way to the right, then to the left, then to the right, etc. Progress is often slow and difficult to assess, but the attendant soon learns to notice that when "new" tissue detaches from the uterus and comes out, it feels warmer than the portion that has been "swinging in the breeze."

3. Infusion of sterile saline solution into the uterus is the next step, based on the premise that the distention of the uterus by the volume of fluid (usually one or two liters) and its saltiness help to alleviate some of the swelling of the villi and crypts and stimulate uterine contraction. The saline has a therapeutic effect as well, helping to dilute the debris and contaminants that accumulate in the uterus after foaling. Specific antibiotics can also be added to the saline as deemed necessary by the veterinarian.

149

4. The final step is to administer oxytocin, which should definitely be done only by a veterinarian since the risk of prolapse is greatest with this approach. The intravenous administration of extremely low doses (20 international units, or 1.0 ml) is best, since the effect is almost immediate, moderate in scale and quickly out of the system. When given by the intravenous (IV) route, oxytocin is out of the system within approximately six minutes after the injection. In most cases, discomfort and sweating are noticeable within two minutes of treatment, and the mare often lies down and works on passing the afterbirth right away. Many veterinarians prefer diluting the oxytocin in a larger volume of sterile saline and administering it by slow IV drip until the desired results are obtained. This has the advantage of lower overall dosage and the capability of stopping treatment as soon as the uterus begins to push the afterbirth out. The only problem with this method is the inconvenience of installing an IV catheter and keeping it properly in position while the mare frets and cramps and lies down in response to the oxytocin. Giving oxytocin intramuscularly (IM) is much less desirable in this situation, since the effects are longer lasting and therefore much more likely to lead to uterine prolapse. The ideal effect is to stimulate uterine contractions just long enough to push out the afterbirth, after which the uterus relaxes and returns to its place in the mare's abdomen.

To delay the decomposition of the afterbirth so that it can be examined later, immerse it in a clean bucket of cool water, and be sure to cover it and place it out of reach of curious dogs and cats. Because of the aforementioned risk of disease transmission, do not allow any horses to have contact with it, especially broodmares, and when you and your veterinarian have finished examining it, dispose of it promptly and according to sanitation ordinances in your area. Common disposal practices include burning the afterbirth, burying it or having it picked up by a service licensed to render animal tissues. To facilitate transferring it to your disposal site, a couple of strong, empty paper feed sacks, one inside the other, make a reliable, temporarily leak-resistant receptacle.

UTERINE PROLAPSE

Besides the hazard of a reluctant afterbirth causing uterine inflammation and infection, there is another more dramatic danger during Stage III that has already been alluded to. It is well known that in the normal situation the uterus pushes the afterbirth out by turning itself inside out. Slowly, gradually, the horns of the uterus evert themselves as they approach the vulva, pushing and detaching the afterbirth along the way. If everything goes according to plan, the afterbirth is completely detached by the time it has been pushed into the birth canal, resulting in the afterbirth falling to the ground in a "shlurp" and the uterus quietly, secretly returning to its normal position in the mare's abdomen. If something goes wrong, however, the uterus may fail to return to the abdomen, instead following the afterbirth out onto the ground. This is called uterine prolapse, and it usually occurs when the last bit of afterbirth is adhered too tightly to the uterus, so that the portion of the afterbirth that has already come out pulls on the portion that is "stuck" to the uterus, pulling the uterus out with it.

Uterine prolapse is also an unfortunate side effect of the injudicious or inappropriate injection of the hormone oxytocin by well-meaning but misguided attendants trying to "help" the mare. Oxytocin (also known as pituitary oxytocic principle, POP, pituitrin or pitocin) causes extremely powerful uterine contractions, and if the injection is given at the wrong time, or if the dosage is too high, or if the mare is especially sensitive to it, her contractions will be too strong and too prolonged, causing the uterus to push itself outside the mare's body. As a general rule, the uterus is more sensitive to oxytocin during the immediate post-foaling period and becomes less sensitive to it as time passes. Many horse breeders and dog breeders have bottles of injectable oxytocin in their possession, although it is difficult to understand why a responsible drug salesman or veterinarian would sell it to them. **The dosage recommendation on the label of most oxytocin preparations is five times higher than can safely be given to a mare, and even when the proper dosage is given, the risk of uterine prolapse is higher than if oxytocin were not given at all.** Therefore it is foolhardy for anyone to administer this substance unless they are trained and prepared to deal with uterine prolapse.

151

Watching a mare until she has passed the afterbirth can be boring and frustrating after the excitement of the foal's birth. Nevertheless, you will be extremely fortunate if all your Stage III vigils are boring. The possibility of uterine prolapse is the most pressing (and anything but boring) reason that you must remain with your mare until the afterbirth has been passed.

Recognizing that a uterine prolapse is occurring is not usually a problem, since the everting uterus looks extremely abnormal even to the inexperienced attendant. Oddly, not all mares will appear to be straining excessively or even to be in any discomfort while in the process of prolapsing the uterus, since abdominal contractions are not necessarily occurring along with the contractions of the uterus itself. Therefore, it is important for the attendant to make an effort to keep an eye on the mare's vulva. The prolapsing uterus is most often described to look initially like an enormous brain protruding from the mare's vulva, and again, this process can be very insidious, **so it's essential that you watch what's happening under the mare's tail.** As the uterus progresses through the vulva, its own weight pulls it down and perpetuates the prolapse. If recognized early, as soon as it begins to protrude, the "big brain" can be pushed back into the mare's vulva relatively easily. Unfortunately, in most cases this will stimulate the mare to push, just as the foal's movements in the mare's vagina stimulate her to push during Stage II.

If the mare pushes now, she will most certainly push the uterus right back at you, and the natural tendency for most attendants is to push back even harder, leaving their hand inside the mare's vagina to keep her from pushing the uterus out. The continued presence of the hand in the vagina merely heightens the mare's reflexive tendency to push, and the situation escalates quickly. The most effective way to stop the mare from prolapsing her uterus is to quickly push it back in, then immediately remove your hand from the vagina and pinch the vulva closed with both hands as though you were pinching your lips, grabbing healthy handfuls of the vulva with your hands. Using this method, the mare's straining usually stops within a few moments, and although it is necessary to remain with her to watch for further attempts to prolapse, in most cases the danger is past.

Have the mare examined by a veterinarian immediately in order to assess the damage and determine whether any further

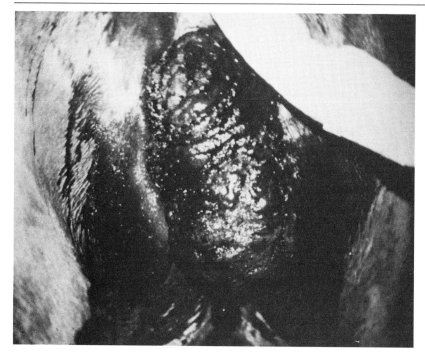

measures should be taken. In most cases, the veterinarian will opt to flush the uterus with appropriate antibiotic-treated solutions and suture the upper part of the vulva closed in an especially tight Caslick's closure in order to prevent immediate recurrence of the prolapse should the mare have prolonged or recurrent contractions. If veterinary attention is delayed, the best way to keep the mare from re-prolapsing after you've pushed the uterus back in is to take her for a brisk walk or trot in-hand with the foal allowed to tag along. Taking her for a stroll down a small hill helps to encourage the uterus to fall forward into the abdomen by taking advantage of gravity. If she wants to stop and strain, do whatever is necessary to get her to trot with you. This serves two purposes: it distracts her from her uterine discomfort, and it also helps to jostle the heavy uterus forward into the lower recesses of the mare's abdomen, from where it will be more difficult for her to heave it out again.

If the prolapse is occurring because it is being pulled out by the weight of an abnormally adhered afterbirth, the afterbirth will have to be detached manually from the uterus before your attempt at replacing the uterus will be effective, since the heavy afterbirth will simply pull the uterus right back out again. This

153

FIGURE 4.73
If (and only if) the pro-
lapse is just beginning,
the informed and pre-
pared attendant can
push it back in relatively
easily, then pull her
hand out and pinch the
lips of the vulva closed
to prevent the mare
from pushing it back out
again. Then, if possible,
take the mare outside
for a downhill trot to
help jostle the uterus
forward.

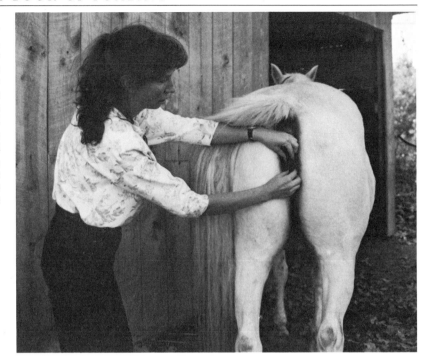

will have to be done without delay, since the prolapse progresses
quickly once it starts.

If you are unlucky enough to have to deal with a uterine
prolapse, **be very careful not to cause any holes or tears in the
uterus,** such as by poking your fingers through it, since this will
have serious and possibly life-threatening consequences. If possible, support the heavy uterus in the palm of one hand and
detach the Velcro-like attachment of the remaining afterbirth
from the spot where it has become too tightly adhered with
your other hand. If the situation is already in the crisis stage, for
example if the afterbirth is too tightly adhered for you to get it
apart from the uterus and the uterus is being pulled out too
quickly by all the weight, you may have to tear the afterbirth (*not* the uterus!) in order to remove the weight before the
uterus comes out too far. **This should be done only if there is no
other alternative.** Try to tear it as close to the uterus as possible
so that the piece of afterbirth that goes back into the mare will
be small, since **this absolutely will cause the uterus to become
infected, it absolutely will require emergency veterinary attention and it may create a very dangerous condition called**

acute endometritis, whereby the mare actually goes into shock. Once again, immediate veterinary attention is *mandatory*. This entire process is best left to the veterinarian, but if you are present when a prolapse starts and there is no veterinarian there to handle it, you should have the knowledge to handle the situation intelligently.

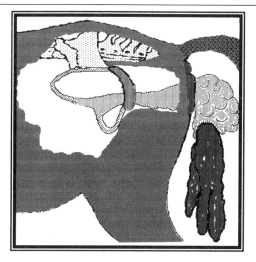

FIGURE 4.74
Some cases of uterine prolapse are caused by a section of afterbirth being inseparably adhered to the uterus. The weight of the heavy afterbirth pulls the uterus out, and in order to halt the prolapse before it comes out all the way, the "stuck" part of the afterbirth will have to be removed or torn while supporting the heavy uterus.

If you find a prolapse already in the advanced stages, already hanging down, do not attempt to replace it without veterinary assistance. You should only push a prolapse back in if you can do so the moment it begins to protrude, before it touches the mare's skin and tail. If the prolapse is already in the more advanced stages, the best thing for you to do is to try and minimize the damage that will occur to the protruding tissues while you await your veterinarian's arrival. In addition to cleaning and replacing the exposed uterine tissue, the veterinarian must ascertain whether the urethra (through which the mare urinates) has been damaged or displaced by the prolapse. This usually requires that the mare's bladder be catheterized aseptically with a sterile mare catheter.

Injury to the uterine tissues will occur from excessive drying, dust, bedding, splinters, filth, flies and physical trauma. By covering it completely with a clean, lightweight cotton bedsheet that has been soaked in clean, clear, cool water, you can help to keep the uterus from drying out and help to slow down the swelling. This sheet should be rinsed out and reapplied periodically, depending on weather conditions and the length of time you must wait for veterinary help. Or, alternately, leave the sheet in place and rewet it periodically with more clean, cool water or with sterile saline solution—which you should always have on hand for irrigating wounds. The goal is to keep the exposed uterus moist and to help keep dirt and bedding from

155

becoming embedded into the crevices of the oozing, swelling tissue. If possible, arrange the sheet like a sling around the uterus so that you can lift the heavy tissue and provide some support for it with the fabric of the sheet, which is tied over the mare's back and secured to the sides of her halter with a jury-rigged rope system.

Flies are a serious problem, because the protruding tissue is everything that a fly could want—it's moist, warm, bloody and inflamed from the traumas of recent birth and the accident of prolapse. In fly season, exposed tissue can become a receptacle for literally thousands of fly eggs in less than an hour's time. **Under no circumstances, however, should you apply any fly repellant or insecticide to the exposed uterine tissue**, since many substances can be absorbed directly into the mare's bloodstream via the raw, oozing uterine lining. Chemical products that are approved for use in horses are meant to be applied to intact skin, and even then, you should take every safety precaution. But when applied to mucosal tissue, such as the exposed lining of the mare's prolapsed uterus, even the most innocuous substances can become deadly poisons. Nothing should touch that tissue except sterile saline, clean fresh water and your clean bedsheet until the veterinarian arrives.

Oddly enough, a mare with a prolapsed uterus usually appears unconcerned with what has happened at her hindquarters and often behaves in a manner that only compounds the trauma. A mare may actually step on her uterus with her own hooves. Her preoccupation with her newborn foal, heightened by the worried presence of humans trying to deal with the prolapse, may make her less likely to stand still for your ministrations and manipulations at her hindquarters, especially if the foal has figured out how to stand up and move around to where the mare can't see him. Many times a mare at this stage of motherhood will be especially concerned with placing herself between the foal and humans, and she may make abrupt or forceful attempts to turn around, flinging her dangling uterus behind her like "crack-the-whip," slapping it against walls, hay racks, water buckets or whatever (and whoever) happens to be in its path. Any forces that serve to further the prolapse, such as added weight on the uterus from the fluid associated with swelling, and such as the centrifugal force associated with rapid turning move-

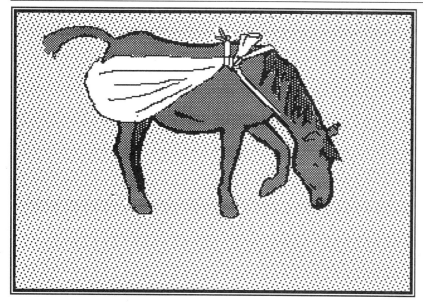

FIGURE 4.75
If the uterine prolapse is already advanced, the damage can be minimized by supporting the heavy, exposed tissues in a clean bedsheet that is kept damp with clean, cool water or sterile saline while waiting for the veterinarian.

ments, should be discouraged as thoroughly and as thoughtfully as possible. Pay attention to detail.

For example, if the mare is concerned because her foal is moving out of view, have someone corral the foal gently and unobtrusively in front of the mare where she can nuzzle and smell him. If the mare is uncomfortable from "afterpains" and seems intent on lying down, try to distract her from the pain by offering a small bran mash or some bite-sized pieces of carrot or apple—not enough food to create a problem if she has a legitimate colic, but enough to get her mind off her aching uterus and to dissuade her from lying down and dragging it through the bedding.

If the mare's agitation seems to be dominating the situation, you may consider having her tranquilized or sedated, but only if your veterinarian agrees. If you are still waiting for veterinary assistance to arrive and you feel it's necessary to give a sedative or tranquilizer to the mare right away, do so only if your veterinarian has given you prior authorization for this particular circumstance, and do so according to the guidelines of the veterinarian's dosage and product recommendations. Be aware that certain types of drugs are better than others in certain situations, and in some cases a usually "safe," commonly used drug may be the *worst* thing to give because of the horse's special situation.

157

For example, while a certain drug may be well known as an effective pain reliever in "colic," that drug may have several side effects, such as causing uterine contractions, slowing down gut motility, lowering blood pressure, increasing stomach acid and ulcers, depressing the respiratory system, increasing urine output and causing the horse to sweat. The term "colic" simply means "bellyache," and many things can cause a bellyache, including fecal impaction, uterine cramping, stomach irritation, ulcers, kidney disease, urinary tract infection, back pain, peritonitis, pleuropneumonia, etc. To the untrained eye, all abdominal pain looks alike, regardless of the cause, and unless you are trained in pharmacology, you would be unlikely to know all the effects of each "common" colic medication. In many cases, one of those side effects could produce disastrous effects if the underlying cause of the colic happens to be something that would be magnified by the side effect. Just because a particular drug is available over the counter at the feed store doesn't mean it's "safe." If you are able to confer with your veterinarian over the telephone about your mare's specific problem before giving any treatments, you will be less likely to give something that will compound the problem. If you are not able to consult your veterinarian, you are much better off staying away from any drug treatments.

After the uterine prolapse crisis has been resolved, the uterus has been cleansed and treated and returned to its proper position, and the condition of the urethra has been assessed, some attention should be given to the mare's milk output and the effect all the hullaballoo may have had on the mare-foal relationship. Mares have been known to "dry up" (halt milk production) after a severe physical insult, particularly when the threat of "blood poisoning" (toxemia) is present. As was previously mentioned, **uterine prolapse leaves the mare at increased risk of acute endometritis, a severe infection of the uterine lining which often leads to toxemia.** This is a possibility that should be taken into account by the attending veterinarian, and medication to prevent infection and toxemia should be instituted immediately. In most cases, the treatment plan will involve certain medications (antibiotics, anti-inflammatories, antihistamines and uterine infusions) that will need to be given for several days. It is important to continue the treatments for the prescribed length of time, since the risk of toxemia is very high during the recovery phase after a uterine prolapse. The veterinarian should consider the effect of the toxins and the prescribed medications on the quality of the mare's milk, and if there is any risk that the foal may be harmed by these factors, steps should be taken to either alter the treatment or to provide the foal with an alternate source of milk until the mare's milk is safe.

If toxemia occurs, a decrease or cessation in milk production is a very real possibility, even if the mare is successfully treated for the toxemia and recovers quickly. Since toxemia is a serious and dramatic condition that can be fatal, it is common for people to concentrate all their concern and attention on the stricken mare at the expense of the foal. In many cases when the mare recovers, she looks so much better (and everyone is so relieved at how healthy and normal she seems after such a traumatic crisis) that it doesn't occur to them that she may not have enough milk now to feed her foal properly. Her udder was full before she became ill—how could she have no milk now? It definitely pays to consider this possibility, because if the foal becomes weak from too little milk at this tender, fragile age, the odds of bringing him back to health with standard, on-site facilities may not be good. For help in determining whether the mare is providing adequate milk, see Section 5.2 on milk production.

RUPTURED UTERINE ARTERY

At the risk of scaring you to death, there is one more disaster that should be discussed in order for this book to prepare you completely for foaling. Rarely, but often enough to warrant discussion, a mare will develop a rip in one of the major arteries leading to the uterus, causing massive internal bleeding. It is often fatal, and although there is no practical way to save the mare, there are a few things you can do to help tip the scales a bit in her favor. But first you have to recognize what's happening.

There are two uterine arteries—one on each side. Each artery resides within a curtain-like ligament called the broad ligament, which hangs from the ceiling of the abdominal cavity, suspending each uterine horn. As the growing pregnancy gets heavier, the broad ligament stretches from the increasing weight, and the artery stretches along with it. With each successive pregnancy the walls of the artery begin to lose elasticity, just as an old rubber band fatigues after repeated use. This paves the way for the artery to rip as the next pregnancy becomes heavier and tugs on the broad ligament. Since the artery is sandwiched between the two layers of the ligament, the initial bleeding is usually restricted to the space between the layers. If the rip is large enough, however, the bleeding is too severe and manages to break through the ligament. The artery then bleeds like a firehose as the blood pours into the free expanses of the abdomen. The mare may actually bleed to death within minutes.

The most common time for this condition to occur is from just before foaling to 24 hours afterwards. The onset is usually sudden with no warning. Statistically there appears to be no relationship between ruptured uterine artery and dystocia—it occurs with equal frequency whether the birthing was easy or difficult because it's the weight, not the contractions, that cause the artery to rip. Therefore, aside from not breeding the mare, there really isn't a whole lot you can do to prevent it. Strenuous exercise during the later stages of pregnancy is obviously not recommended, since this may bounce the heavy uterus, stressing the groaning ligament and its already stretched-to-the-limit artery. Once it occurs, however, quick action may increase the odds that the mare will survive—this is another situation where having the veterinarian on the scene at the start of every foaling will ensure that professional help is there when it is needed most.

Internal bleeding is painful—the blood irritates the tissues lining the abdominal cavity and organs and creates pain. The more blood, and the faster it comes, the greater the pain. A mare that is bleeding internally looks as though she's having a severe bout with colic, thrashing and rolling violently. The biggest mistake at this point would be to try to get the mare on her feet, since this would only increase her blood pressure and make her bleed faster. Instead, get the foal out of the stall and out of harm's way, and once the diagnosis of hemorrhage has been made, the mare should be treated with a strong painkiller with sedative effects, which will have the happy side effect of lowering her blood pressure. Most veterinarians choose the sedative xylazine, which is one of the strongest abdominal pain medications with profound effects on the blood pressure. Unless the hemorrhaging is too rapid or advanced, the heavily sedated mare will lie quietly and sleep hard, usually snoring, for several hours. Hopefully she will sleep long enough to form a secure blood clot over the rip. Surgery is rarely feasible, since the patient is an abysmal anesthetic risk, and since transporting the mare to the hospital would almost surely be fatal.

While the mare sleeps, much attention should be focused on the foal, since he is likely to be orphaned. Take as much colostrum from the mare as you can, giving the proper amounts to the foal at the proper intervals and storing the rest in the freezer as described in Section 5.1.

If the mare awakens, all efforts should focus on keeping her calm and severely restricting her movements, since an increase in blood pressure may blow the blood clot and start the hemorrhaging all over again. Rebreeding her down the line is a decision that should be made after much soul-searching, since she is a prime candidate to hemorrhage again. The odds of surviving a single hemorrhage are low enough—the odds of surviving a second episode are not even worth mentioning.

One of the most important things to understand about ruptured uterine artery is that, aside from breeding the mare, nothing you did caused the rupture to happen—it wasn't your fault. Furthermore, if it occurs, there isn't a blessed thing you can do about it except try to encourage clotting by keeping the mare calm and quiet and lowering her blood pressure. The odds are against her, so you must be realistic and take steps to prepare your new foal for life without his mother.

Section 4.8

Important Deworming

Research at the University of Illinois Veterinary Medical Teaching Hospital in 1988 revealed that treatment of mares within twelve hours of parturition with oral ivermectin can prevent the development of certain intestinal parasites in their foals. Subsequent studies upheld the report, indicating that the ivermectin treatment essentially provided foals with an opportunity for a lifetime free of infestation by the parasite *Strongyloides westeri*.

Until this discovery, foals had been subject to the same old game of "catch-up" whereby they were ensured of initial infestation, followed by treatment, followed by reinfestation and re-treatment, etc. With the immediate post-foaling ivermectin treatment of their dams, however, and if the foals themselves are given regular follow-up deworming treatments in concert with good hygiene, uncrowded pasturing and at least twice weekly manure pickup to prevent seeding of the environment with infectious eggs from other infested horses, they can actually look forward to a worm-free life, at least where this particular kind of worm is concerned.

According to the study, the timing of the treatment is crucial. Treatment after 12 hours of birth, as well as the use of any deworming product other than ivermectin* will not yield the reported results. Since ivermectin is approved for use in pregnant mares and in very young foals, and since the implications of the report are so important, it seems foolhardy not to follow the recommendations of the study. A lifetime free of *Strongyloides westeri* infection can mean total exemption from the damage these parasites normally inflict during their hike through the internal organs and may mean less worm-related colic in the lifetime of the foal.

Another concept that bears further investigation is the use of daily dewormers in horses, particularly broodmares during pregnancy and while lactating. Recent research has shown that the daily use of the dewormer pyrantel tartate† essentially breaks the lifecycle of many intestinal parasites before they can damage the horse's intestines and blood vessels and before certain of the eggs can be shed in a mare's milk to infect her nursing foal.

---

* *Eqvalan and Zimectrin, Merck Sharp and Dohme Laboratories.*
† *Strongid-C pelleted daily dewormer, Pfizer Pharmaceuticals.*

BABY'S FIRST 12 HOURS

Section 5.1
Colostrum

The foal's intestinal system is designed to be especially absorbent during the first 12 hours of life. This allows the antibodies that are present in the mare's colostrum to be absorbed into the foal's bloodstream so that he will have some protection against disease until his immune system is able to build antibodies of its own. Antibodies are particularly large molecules that would ordinarily not be absorbed by the intestinal tract, and the ability of the newborn foal's intestines to absorb these large molecules is temporary and very short-lived. Research has shown that peak absorption of antibody-rich colostrum occurs at about 3 hours. Therefore, it is important that the foal's first several meals consist of an adequate quantity and quality of colostrum. This is a concept that seems to be relatively well understood by the horse industry.

The protection afforded the foal by the colostrum is primarily in the form of a protein immunoglobulin known as immunoglobulin-G, or IgG. Colostrum differs from "regular" milk in other ways as well, however, including energy and fat content and physical appearance. It is not possible to judge the quality (antibody content) of the colostrum simply by virtue of its thick, rich appearance. Yet the strict time constraints placed on the ingestion of colostrum make it especially important that the foal receive nothing but very good quality colostrum during those crucial first hours—**it is not advisable to allow the three-hour-old foal to take poor-quality colostrum or "regular" milk tonight in the hope that you'll be able to find better colostrum for him tomorrow.** Furthermore, it should never be assumed that the foal's natural mother, with her ample udder and voluminous supply of milk, is necessarily providing the foal with colostrum which optimally protects him against disease. It is not uncommon for a perfectly healthy mare to give her newborn foal oodles of milk that is deficient in antibody protection. Therefore, it is a very good idea to test the quality of the colostrum as soon as the foal is born so that an alternate source of protection can be provided right away if necessary.

Laboratory assessment of IgG content in colostrum can be expensive and difficult to obtain, especially at three o'clock in the morning. Techniques used in the laboratory to measure IgG can be quite technical and may not be readily available in remote or rural areas. Because most foalings occur in the middle of the night and since foals should receive their colostrum within 8 to 12 hours, evaluation of equine colostrum ideally should be done on site using an easy and readily available technique that anyone can learn to do. Research has shown that the *specific gravity* of the colostrum closely correlates with its IgG content, and a crude but adequately accurate assessment of colostral specific gravity can be taken easily on farm, requiring minimal instruction and equipment.

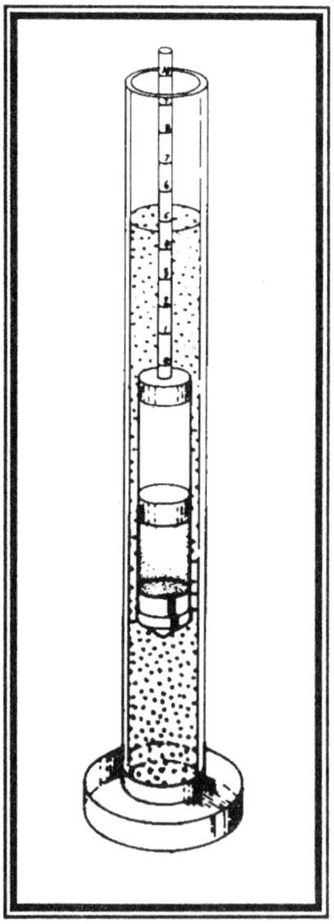

The Equine Colostrometer (Jorgenson Manufacturing, Loveland, Colorado) is a widely accepted instrument used for

FIGURE 5.01
The Equine Colostrometer, available from Jorgenson Manufacturing of Loveland, Colorado, can be used in the field to measure specific gravity of colostrum.

164

on-farm measurement of colostral specific gravity. The device comes with instructions, which must be followed closely, but the procedure is not difficult and takes less than 5 minutes to complete.

A slightly less accurate (but usually adequate) method for testing specific gravity of colostrum involves the use of a hand-held instrument called a clinical refractometer. Field use of the refractometer has yielded measurements that closely correlate with the measurements obtained from the Colostrometer, with the added benefit of requiring less than 10 seconds and absolutely no setup. Since the refractometer, which can be obtained from laboratory supply distributors,does not always come with instructions for proper use, and since its use for assessment of colostrum is not widely accepted as yet, a brief description of its proper use in this regard follows.

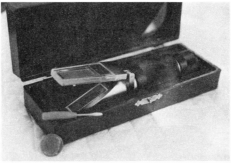

FIGURE 5.02
The hand-held clinical refractometer can be used to assess the specific gravity of colostrum.

By definition, the specific gravity of a substance is the ratio of the weight of that substance compared to the weight of an equal volume of another substance (usually water). Most of us think of measuring weights by using a scale, but in the case of colostrum, we're really not interested in what the colostrum *weighs*—we're only interested in the weight *ratio* of colostrum to water. The clinical refractometer measures that ratio directly, and it works on the premise that a drop of liquid of high specific gravity will be more difficult to compress than will a drop of liquid with a lower specific gravity.

To calibrate the device, clean the working surface with distilled water and wipe it dry with a lint-free cloth. Place a drop of distilled water in the

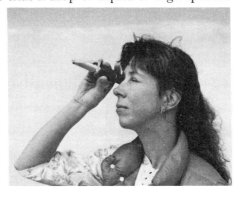

FIGURE 5.03
The refractometer is "read" by holding it up to the light and looking into the eyepiece, revealing a tiny scale of numbers superimposed over a "horizon." Where the horizon intersects with the scale is the specific gravity.

center of the "window" with a medicine dropper, and lower the plastic "lid" onto the drop of water. Then hold the eyepiece of the refractometer up to one eye like a telescope and aim it at a bright light, revealing a scale similar to the one shown in Figure 5.04. Since specific gravity is most often measured in urine samples in medical practice, the specific gravity scale on many clinical refractometers is labeled U.G., for "urine gravity." This is

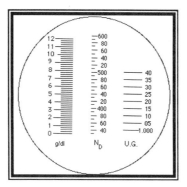

FIGURE 5.04
A typical refractometer will have from 1 to 3 scales. The SG or specific gravity scale (also referred to as urine gravity, or UG) is the one used for colostrum.

the scale we're interested in. Notice that the scale is superimposed on a background that consists of a white "sea" and a blue "sky." The horizon, where the sea and sky meet, is where the scale is read. It is known by convention that the specific gravity of distilled water is 1.000, and if the horizon is not exactly on the 1.000 mark, the refractometer should be adjusted (calibrated) so that it reads the proper specific gravity for water. The calibration screw is located on the top of the device, and a tiny screwdriver (which usually comes with the refractometer when purchased) is used to turn the screw while looking through the eyepiece until the horizon crosses the scale at 1.000.

After you've calibrated the refractometer, wipe the working surface dry with a lint-free cloth or lens paper, place one drop of fresh colostrum in the center of the window and lower the lid. This time the horizon should intersect the scale much higher, preferably at or above 1.080 ("ten-eighty"). Exceptionally good

FIGURE 5.05
Specific gravity of three different colostrum samples:
A: 1.040
B: 1.055
C: off the scale
Note that each field (circle) contains three scales. Ignore the first two. Read only the scale on the right.

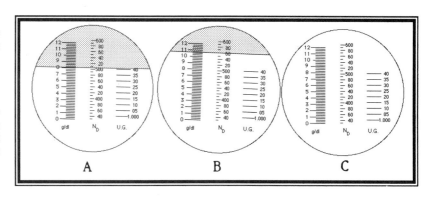

A   B   C

colostrum will have a specific gravity so high that the horizon is off the scale, such that you'll see no blue "sky," only white "sea." The specific gravity scales of many refractometers don't go higher than 1.040 ("ten-forty"), but with practice the number can be guessed quite easily. When you're finished reading the specific gravity of the colostrum, be sure to clean and dry the window and lid of the refractometer thoroughly with distilled water and a clean, lint-free cloth or lens paper. Store it in its container in a safe place until the next foaling.

If the specific gravity of the colostrum is lower than 1.060 ("ten-sixty"), the foal should be supplemented with better colostrum. As a rule of thumb, a normal foal should receive at least 30 ounces of colostrum with a specific gravity of 1.070 or above by the time he's 8 hours old.

In addition to providing a means by which the foal can receive protective antibodies, it should be understood that the temporarily heightened absorbency of the newborn foal's intestinal tract also leaves the foal exceptionally vulnerable to the effects of absorbing *other* substances, which may be *harmful* to his health. Bear in mind that if the mare has just been through a toxic disease process, the infectious organisms, their toxins, and any medications that were administered to the mare may now be present in her milk. If the possibility of tainted milk exists, there are two important problems which must be addressed.

FINDING AN ALTERNATE SOURCE OF COLOSTRUM

First, an alternate source of good-quality (specific gravity of 1.080 or above) horse colostrum must be obtained. **Cow colostrum, goat colostrum or colostrum from any other species than a horse is not appropriate**, since the antibodies contained in the colostrum of other species will not provide protection against most *horse* diseases. It is generally agreed that the newborn foal should receive at least 30 ounces of good-quality colostrum during its first 8 to 12 hours of life, and the sooner the better, because with each passing hour the intestinal tract is closing its doors to the larger molecules. Remember, optimal absorption occurs at 3 hours.

Plan ahead to have colostrum available in case your mare is unable to provide safe, good-quality colostrum of her own. Some

167

equine veterinarians keep a few ounces of horse colostrum in their freezers, but it is generally not feasible for them to maintain a current colostrum bank. Some of the larger breeding farms do maintain colostrum banks, and they are usually more than happy to share some of their stock with a fellow horseman. Additionally, some of the more progressive horse enthusiast associations maintain colostrum banks, and in many cases colostrum is made available to individuals free of charge as long as it is replaced with good-quality colostrum from another mare as soon as possible. If several sources are available, it is usually possible to beg enough colostrum from each source to accumulate the recommended 30 ounces. There are also commercial colostrum banks that are in the business of stockpiling and selling colostrum, and their product is usually tested for quality and dated. Rather than rely on others to provide you with colostrum at the last panic-stricken moment, the best policy is to locate and contact a commercial colostrum bank and purchase the requisite 30 ounces *before* your mare's foaling date so that it will be in your freezer in case of need. Then, if it turns out that you didn't need it, you can share it with other breeders.

The newborn foal's stomach is small, and although it gradually stretches to accommodate gradually increasing volumes, its capacity is initially restricted to less than 12 ounces. Unfortunately, young foals often fail to regulate their intake and can get a whale of a bellyache if they drink too much too fast. In the natural situation, when the foal is nursing from the mare, there is no practical way to measure and regulate the volume of milk the foal suckles. However, the rate of flow of milk from the mare's udder is usually slow enough to allow the foal to "feel full" before he drinks too much.

When giving colostrum from a baby bottle, however, the rate of flow is only crudely regulated. A nipple with only a pinpoint opening will provide too little milk and too little reinforcement for continued suckling effort. Enlarging the hole will allow the milk to flow more freely, but if the hole is too large, a foal can drain a 12-ounce bottle in less than a minute, almost surely resulting in discomfort. **The rule of thumb should be to mimic the natural situation as closely as possible, which is to provide small, frequent meals.**

If bottle feeding is necessary, therefore, limit the newborn's bottle feedings to 6 to 8 ounces per hour, and if time permits, feed 4 ounces every 30 minutes instead. If the entire colostrum dosage of 30 ounces must be given by bottle, strive to have the 30 ounces into the foal by his eighth hour of life or sooner, giving *no more* than 8 ounces per hour. This gives you plenty of time to get the minimum amount of colostrum into the foal, and if more than 30 ounces are available, that's great—there's always more time. If using frozen colostrum, be sure to thaw only the amount needed for the immediate feeding, since it doesn't "keep" well after thawing.

Frozen colostrum is fragile with respect to its quality. If improperly thawed or overheated, the antibodies in it will be ruined and the colostrum will be no more valuable than regular milk. Colostrum is best thawed slowly, immersed in its container into a bowl of cool water until it is thawed, then placed in water that is slightly warmer until the milk itself has reached a temperature that is slightly cooler than body temperature. If a thermometer is available, the colostrum should be warmed to about 98° F. When in doubt, it would be better to have it too cool rather than too warm, since the IgG antibodies in overheated colostrum are damaged, and since overheated milk in general tends to cause foal diarrhea. To avoid wasting valuable colostrum, it should be offered to the foal in a baby bottle using the technique described in Section 5.3.

Special note: Colostrum should always be handled and stored in very clean plastic containers, since reports indicate that the protein antibodies in the colostrum are degraded upon contact with glass.

If the mare's colostrum is good quality, it is good policy to save some of it for future need. If the foal is at least 8 hours old and has been nursing well from his dam, or if you have been giving bottled colostrum and are sure that he has received at least 30 ounces by the eighth hour of life, it is reasonable to begin "stealing" a total of 8 to 12 ounces of colostrum from the mare at this point to store in your freezer. Colostrum with a specific gravity of 1.090 or greater is generally considered suitable for banking. The most convenient method is to freeze individual 4- to 6-ounce aliquots of colostrum in their own sterile baby bottle (without the nipple). The nipples should be stored separately, since the rubber does not tolerate freezing very well. An alternate method is to use clean zip-top plastic bags made for freezer storage, evacuating excess air out of the bags before sealing the tops. Although it's a clever system, freezing the colostrum in ice cube trays is not advised unless the trays are very clean and are placed in clean, freezer-grade plastic bags before entering the freezer. Once frozen, the individual colostrum cubes can be transferred out of the tray into freezer bags. However, if your freezer is a "frost-free" model, the cubes will probably melt a little bit during the defrost cycles, and when you need three or four cubes for the foal's next colostrum meal, you may be frustrated to find that they're all frozen together. Furthermore, the repeated partial melting and refreezing associated with frost-free freezers dramatically shortens the lifespan of the colostrum's antibodies. If properly handled and kept frozen without interruption, good colostrum can be kept for up to two years.

MANUAL MILKING AND TAINTED MILK

The second problem which must be addressed if your mare has tainted milk is to assure that she will continue to make milk after the problems are resolved. This requires that you manually milk the mare's udder every 2 hours. If your technique is thoughtful and gentle, you should meet with little or no resistance from the mare and you should be able to "empty" the udder completely at each milking. The milk should be discarded responsibly until it is no longer potentially dangerous to the foal, at which time the foal can be returned to its dam to resume natural nursing.

The manufacture of milk within the udder is controlled by (1) hormonal input, (2) the presence or absence of the physical suckling stimulus and (3) the amount of pressure within the udder. If the hormonal environment is normal and has not been altered by external factors such as fever, disease processes, toxins, medications or extreme stress, the normal initiation of milk production should be in progress. The normal hormonal environment will signal for continued milk production as long as the physical environment provides the proper cues.

If, for example, the foal is weak or dead or otherwise prevented from nursing, the mare's teats will be deprived of external stimulation. The stimulation of the teats normally causes the release of oxytocin from the pituitary gland at the base of the mare's brain, and the udder responds to the oxytocin by "opening the floodgates," allowing the milk that is sequestered in its ducts to be released through the teats. This process is called "milk letdown." Additionally, if the foal is not nursing, the

Special note: For information on obtaining colostrum, or to contribute colostrum to the bank, contact:

ENEP / Colostrum Network

CVM, LACS, Dept 225
Teaching Hospital
1365 Gortner Ave
St Paul, MN 55108
(612) 647-8391

udder will become excessively full of milk, since the milk is produced continuously in spite of the fact that the foal is not removing any of it by suckling. The increased pressure within the bulging udder will eventually create negative feedback to the milk-producing glands, resulting in a decrease and eventually a cessation in milk production. This is the same process that allows the mare to "dry up" after weaning.

Section 5.2
Milk Production

It is difficult to assess the volume of milk a foal gets from a nursing session, since he may make audible sucking and swallowing noises even if he is only getting a small dribble of milk for his efforts. Most mares will permit you to milk them manually into a container, thus enabling you to measure the volume of milk being produced in a given length of time. However, the process of milk letdown is, to a degree, under the "conscious" control of the mare, to the extent that if she is agitated, in pain, distrustful, or otherwise unhappy about your efforts to milk her, she may be able to block the release of oxytocin and prevent or abbreviate milk letdown. Some mares will produce and let down so much milk for the suckling foal that one teat is squirting milk up his nostril while he is suckling on the other one, and yet these same mares may provide a paltry one or two ounces for the human milker and then stubbornly shut down.

It could be tempting at this point to force milk letdown by giving an injection of oxytocin to the mare, but two important factors should convince you not to do this indiscriminately. First, this should only be done by a veterinarian, since the oxytocin will cause uterine contractions that could result in a uterine prolapse if the uterus is still up in the birth canal at the time of the injection. Secondly, oxytocin causes unpleasant side effects, and the abdominal discomfort associated with it may cause the mare to resent manipulation of her udder, and she may even link the manipulation of her udder with the abdominal pain, as though one caused the other. This could create an aversive conditioning response similar to some of the more rad-

Special note: Mares that are reluctant to let down their milk for human hands may acquiesce after their tense, full udders have been softened and relaxed by a five-minute treatment with a warm, moist towel and a gentle massage. An occasional upward nudge (gently!) with the hand may also simulate the actions of a suckling foal and convince the mare to let down.

ical methods utilized by "stop smoking" clinics, whereby smoking a cigarette becomes mentally linked with electric shocks or nausea or some other unpleasant effect. It may seem far-fetched to suggest that the maternal instinct of allowing one's offspring to suckle can be blocked by the side effect of a medication, but some maiden mares are quite tentative in their acceptance of a newborn foal's advances, and in some cases the addition of one more aversive stimulus can be the last straw in the mare's "decision" to behave aggressively toward the foal.

Although definitely lacking in objectivity, the most consistent (and obviously less invasive) method of assessing the volume of milk the foal is getting is to watch the mare and foal for some specific clues. Once the foal has successfully located the mare's teats and has managed to keep a teat in his mouth long enough to receive a milk reward, the mare's behavior may be used as one indicator of the adequacy of the foal's meals. Many mares will initially resent the clumsy and sometimes brutal bumping of their tender, swollen udders by the foal's muzzle. It appears that prior to the first good nursing, the udder is so swollen and sore that even the gentlest touch is painful. However, once the foal has "latched on" to a teat and has initiated a significant flow of milk, the mare usually appears relieved, as though the streaming of milk through the teat alleviates the pain and actually provides some pleasure. The anxious expression in the mare's eyes usually softens and she begins to take on a glazed, almost hypnotized appearance. By the same token, most foals become suddenly sleepy after taking a satisfying milk meal, and if your foal lies down and sleeps deeply for 10 to 30 minutes after nursing, it is likely that he is getting plenty of milk.

On the other hand, if for some reason the foal's suckling efforts do not result in a significant flow of milk, he will continue to pester the mare, rarely stopping for a long nap. The mare may begin to resent his presence, and his persistent suckling and bumping will be met with an escalation of her displeasure as the teats and udder become increasingly irritated, with none of the pleasant sensations associated with normal milk letdown. As the situation deteriorates, the mare-foal relationship erodes, and before long the foal may be in danger of being bitten or kicked by his previously protective dam. It is reasonably safe to assume at this stage that the foal is *not* receiving adequate milk to satiate

Special Note: Normal neonatal foals nurse an average of three to seven times per hour. If nursing more often, consider the possibility that they're not getting enough milk. If the mare's udder is too full, the foal may be ill or weak and in need of veterinary assistance.

Special Note: If the mare still hasn't passed the afterbirth, she may be preoccupied with the associated discomfort. Also, when the afterbirth finally does pass, natural release of oxytocin is involved, which may lead to better milk letdown.

his hunger, and steps should be taken to determine whether this is simply the result of a grouchy, sore mare or whether there is a problem with milk production and/or milk letdown.

Section 5.3
The Aggressive Mare

In some cases, particularly when the mare is new to motherhood, the problem is simply a matter of inexperience on the mare's part. She may be overwhelmed by the processes she has endured: the incredible pain, the dramatic foaling, the physical and emotional intrusion by humans, the physical and emotional intrusion by this strange (but strangely familiar) foal, and his painful and insulting battering of her aching udder. Most of these cases, however, respond favorably to thoughtful and gentle "counseling" by a trusted human. If you suspect that your mare is threatening to harm her hungry newborn, your efforts should focus on (1) protecting the foal, (2) getting a nourishing dose of colostrum into his system and (3) modifying the mare's attitude and behavior so that the conflict will not continue. This usually requires a delicate balance of restraint at the mare's halter, positive reinforcement when she allows the foal to approach and touch her, and negative reinforcement and/or punishment when she behaves aggressively toward the foal.

Everybody is tired at this point, and it is easy for tempers to be short. Patience, gentleness and fortitude are needed to coax the mare into accepting the foal's advances. In many cases, her behavior appears to be a classic love-hate process, whereby she's worried and possessive about the foal but threatens to bite or kick when he approaches. Getting angry and exasperated with her for her bad behavior may only escalate her anxiety and make the negative association with the foal even more deeply rooted. To make matters more complicated, in some cases human interference tends to make the mare more anxious and irritable, and her increasingly hostile treatment of the foal may be a manifestation of displaced aggression. **Each situation is different and must be assessed moment by moment.** If you determine that human intervention is necessary to protect the foal and fortify

173

the mare-foal relationship, be as noninvasive as possible. Once again, extraneous noise and extra personnel should be eliminated from the nursery area.

If it seems necessary to apply additional restraint to the mare, the use of the "nose twitch" should be avoided. Although the twitch is effective in selected cases, it has been shown to cause an increase in blood pressure, which could result in increased hemorrhage in the mare's raw reproductive tract and birth canal. It is generally more effective to distract the mare with such diversions as bite-sized pieces of carrot or apple (given sparingly and at strategic times). Sometimes a gentle, rhythmic tapping on the center of the mare's forehead has a calming, distracting, almost hypnotic effect. Gently touching the inner corner (medial canthus) of the mare's eyes is also effective in some cases. Many horses appreciate being scratched in their favorite itchy places, such as on the forehead, behind the ears, between the front legs and on the withers. Providing the mare with one or more of these pleasant diversions while she is behaving well, then obviously removing the reward (with or without the addition of a sharp word or slap on the side of the neck) when her behavior is unacceptable, should get the message across that it's profitable to behave well and unprofitable (and sometimes costly) to behave badly. If all the tricks have been used and the mare's behavior is still deplorable, the use of a sedative or tranquilizer may be warranted. The most commonly used agents are acepromazine, xylazine, detomidine and diazepam. The choice of medication should be made by the veterinarian, since some agents may "leak" into the milk and have some effect on the foal. Furthermore, certain types of behavior may be made worse by some drugs—fear, for example, may be elevated to frenzy in some individuals who are sensitive to phenothiazine-type tranquilizers (such as acepromazine).

On some occasions when the mare displays aggressive behavior while the foal is still only an hour or two old, dramatic results can be achieved by draping the afterbirth over the foal's back. This appears to have the effect of strengthening the olfactory (smell) recognizability of the foal to the mare, as though he did not smell "familiar" prior to donning his coat made of afterbirth. In truth, the aggressive mare's behavior resembles that of a normal mare reacting to being approached by somebody else's foal. Statistically, the incidence of foal rejection by maiden mares is increased significantly when the afterbirth is removed from the stall within an hour of the foaling, which may be cause to rethink the earlier recommendation in this book (page 145) to remove it from the stall as soon as it comes out. As always, consider each case individually, especially when the mare is a first-time mother.

In many cases, the mare may have perfectly normal maternal instincts, but her low tolerance for pain has brought the aching in her uterus and udder to the forefront of her consciousness, and the foal's clumsy bumping and nudging are simply too much to bear. In nature, the mare and foal are not confined to a stall or paddock, and the mare is forced to walk and trot in order to keep her youngster in tow. The exercise is often therapeutic, both physiologically and in terms of providing a distraction. In domesticated life, however, free-ranging space is not always available, so the mare may not have the luxury of "walking out the kinks." The stall walls also make it more difficult for the mare to escape the persistent attempts of the foal, and she may resort to aggression as her only option to avoid additional pain. Although in nature it may be feasible to postpone suckling until the mare naturally recovers from her post-foaling aches and pains, the increased risk of exposure to disease in concentrated stable conditions makes it important to get the foal nursing earlier than might be the case in the wild in order to get those essential antibodies. Furthermore, some mares are more sensitive to pain than others, and relief is easily and safely at hand. In these cases, dramatic results are often achieved with a very light one-time dose (75 mg, or 1.5cc intravenously) of flunixin meglumine.* Relief from the pain occurs within fifteen minutes, and improvement in the mare-foal relationship seems to occur simultaneously.

If it appears that the mare may permanently reject the foal, efforts to persuade her to accept him may include keeping her tranquilized, usually with acepromazine, for several days. This should not be undertaken without a full appreciation of the potential side effects and the efforts that must be taken to coun-

Special Note: When figuring dosages, many people are confused by the terminology. A "cc" (which stands for "cubic centimeter") is the same as an "ml" (which stands for "milliliter").

---

* Banamine, Schering Corporation, Kenilworth, New Jersey.

teract the negative effects of the treatment. For example, a tranquilized mare will not move around as much as a normal mare. In the normal situation, the birth fluids that remain in the uterus are encouraged to "slosh out" when the mare trots around to keep up with her foal. Mares that are confined to stalls are already at increased risk of prolonged uterine cramping and possible infection because of the limited exercise they get in their stalls. If the mare is tranquilized, all external functions tend to slow down, including motor movement, eating, drinking, urinating and defecating. Therefore, special attention should be given to forcing exercise in mares that are confined and/or tranquilized.

An easy and effective method is to take the mare and foal for a walk outside the stall. In most cases the foal will follow willingly as long as the mare is not too far away. If a clean paddock or small pasture is available for their exclusive use, and if the weather is cooperative, turning the mare and foal out for free exercise often does wonders for the mare's psychological and physical health. In fact, some mares that appear to reject their foals while confined to a stall will suddenly become exemplary mothers when turned out into a larger area, showing no displeasure at the foal's approach and even allowing him to nurse at will. In many cases returning them to the stall is accompanied by a return of the sour disposition, as though the mare becomes claustrophobic when confined to close quarters with the foal.

Various methods of keeping the mare and foal separated from each other have been used to assure the safety of foals with aggressive mothers, and sometimes these methods actually work toward resolving the mare's behavior problem. The idea is to separate the mare and foal enough to prevent the mare from harming the foal but not enough to allow them to become "psychologically weaned" from each other. The foal should have access to the mare's udder without being exposed to her kicks and bites.

One method involves confining the mare to one end of the stall in such a manner that she can move forward and backward, but she can't turn around. The barrier is a beam or pole that is placed strategically at a height that allows access to the udder but which restricts the mare's lateral kicking efforts and prevents biting by restricting lateral flexibility. With this method, the foal has unlimited access to the mare, whether she likes it or not. If claustrophobia is the mare's problem, this method is apt to "make or break" the mare and may *heighten* her resentment of the foal. Since restriction of her movements is an integral part of this method, special attention must be paid to her physical and psychological needs to get out and move around. An additional drawback to this method is the fact that the mare is restricted from lying down. In many cases this method seems excessive and too closely resembles punishment to be warranted. However, if less extreme methods are ineffective, this may be the only way to avoid hand-rearing the foal.

Another method is to build a low barrier to confine the *foal* to a portion of the stall where the mare can approach and nuzzle him but he can't get out and approach the mare. If the mare is "claustrophobic," this method allows her to have some private time without constantly being harassed by the foal, and the foal, requiring much less space than his mother, seems content with his confinement as long as he can see her. Every hour the mare is held by the halter and encouraged to stand while the foal is released from his pen and allowed to approach the mare and nurse. The foal soon learns to drink enough milk to satisfy his hunger until the next hourly feeding.

If the mare is actually vicious with the foal and behaves aggressively toward him even when he is "minding his own business," careful consideration should be given to raising him as an orphan. Research has suggested that some overly aggressive mares will "soften" toward their foals when treated with altrenogest (Regumate) orally, but constant vigilance is necessary until the foal's safety is reasonably assured, and the effect of such treatment on milk production has yet to be determined. In most cases, if a mare's behavior toward her foal indicates that she lacks sufficient maternal instinct and there are no extenuating circumstances to explain or excuse her behavior, the pattern tends to repeat itself with subsequent foalings and the mare can be expected to be a "foal rejector" every year. The cause of this abnormal behavior has not been studied adequately to say whether it is consistently due to inadequate, excessive or unbalanced hormonal influences, mental deficiencies, learning disabilities, experience or other factors. It is possible that several factors apply. There is no doubt that human intervention can actually cause some mares to behave aggressively toward their young, and many of these mares can be salvaged for subsequent foalings if management practices are improved. Skilled behavior modification techniques combined with trial and error have successfully rehabilitated some mares over a period of two or three foalings, suggesting that in these cases the mares had initially "learned" to be poor mothers. As a rule of thumb, if removing the foal from the mare's immediate area does not elicit an anxious response on the mare's part, the chances of stimulating her to have normal maternal behavior are very slim.

Sometimes all that is needed is some relief from the pressure on the mare's overfull udder. In this case, milk letdown is usually not a problem as long as the mare can be coaxed into standing still and tolerating manipulation of her teats. A simple solution to this situation is to hand-milk the mare yourself, assuming that your technique is effective and gentle. Remember what you learned earlier in the section on testing the mare's milk before foaling (Section 1.3)—do not "strip" the nipple with your fingers, since this is irritating and will be very unpleasant for an already sensitive and swollen teat. Remember also what you learned about preventing future foal diarrhea—research has shown that if the udder is gently washed and rinsed before the foal's first meal, the incidence of foal diarrhea is significantly reduced. And don't lubricate your fingers with saliva before milking the mare! Furthermore, a gentle washing and rinsing with warm water, a soft cloth, and a gentle hand may be much appreciated by the mare and may serve to soften her turgid teats. An added advantage is that after giving this warm sponge bath, your hands will also be clean and warm and less irritating to the mare.

WASHING THE UDDER
Be considerate in your approach of the mare's udder, working your way to it gradually if necessary, demonstrating by your actions that you will be gentle and careful in your handling of the sensitive tissues. Once you have gained access to the udder itself, apply the warm, wet, soft washcloth to the udder and hold it there, without rubbing, the way a barber would soften a man's beard before lathering and shaving. Do this for several minutes,

refreshing the washcloth with more warm water periodically, squeezing enough of the water out of the cloth so that it doesn't irritate the mare by dripping on her hind limbs. When the mare seems relaxed, begin washing the udder, using only a few drops of Ivory liquid soap (not detergent), which you have warmed in your hands, massaging it into a thin lather over the entire udder and between its two halves. Finally, incorporate the nipples in the lathering. When the udder is well lathered, begin rinsing, switching to a fresh bucket of warm water if necessary, until all traces of soap have been removed. Dab the excess water off with a soft hand towel, and prepare to milk the mare.

MILKING THE MARE

Try to find a comfortable yet safe position for yourself while milking the mare, since even the most profuse milkers seem to take forever to produce enough milk to meet your needs. In reality it doesn't take that long, but your arms, back and neck may begin to ache from the effort anyway. Don't become complacent in believing that the mare can be trusted while you are milking her—she probably *can* be trusted, but one swift kick or sidestep can leave you seriously injured if you aren't able to get out of the way fast enough. It's always better to be prepared. To review safe milking technique, see Milking Safety in Section 1.3.

The best container in which to express the mare's milk is a sterile, wide-mouthed container that has a handle. Choose one that is easily cleaned and is relatively lightweight. A see-through plastic 4-cup kitchen measuring cup is

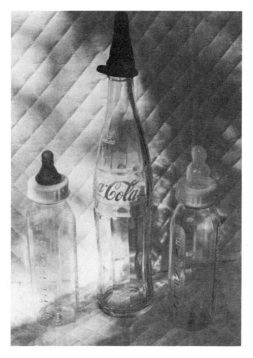

FIGURE 5.06
Some of the more successful setups for bottle feeding a newborn foal include the standard human baby bottle, a black rubber sheep's nipple on a clean soda bottle, and the contemporary-style human baby bottle with the "NUK" nipple.

179

the right size and shape for this task, since the wide opening makes it easy to guide the streams of milk into the container, and since it is also helpful to be able to see at a glance how much milk you have. It is not uncommon, while you are milking one teat, for milk to stream out of the opposite teat at the same time. If the opening of your container is wide enough, you can catch both streams and avoid wasting valuable colostrum. It is generally more efficient to work on milking one side of the udder until it is "empty" before switching to the other teat. Don't milk both sides at the same time, and don't set the milk container on the ground where a careless hoof could knock it over and waste what you've collected.

Even a small Arabian mare should be producing at least 8 ounces of milk every hour (4 ounces from each side) during the first couple of days after foaling. However, even if the mare seems willing and able to give you more than 8 ounces, the foal should not drink more than 8 ounces at a time for his first few meals, since stomach upset can result from overfeeding. Therefore, if it is your intention to give this milk to the foal, try to take 4 ounces from each side, and then quit. The milk that remains in the udder will "keep" much better in the udder than in your refrigerator or anyplace else. (If, on the other hand, the mare is producing so much milk that it is streaming onto the ground between milking sessions, take some of the excess out of the udder and store it in the freezer for future use rather than allow it to be wasted.) Being careful not to spill any of the valuable colostrum, pour it into a sterile baby bottle. If it has any foreign matter such as hair or dirt in it, you may want to pour it through a piece of clean cheesecloth to filter it. Apply the nipple and cap, then check to be sure the hole at the end of the nipple is large enough for milk to spill out freely in drips (not in a stream) when you tilt the bottle. If the hole needs to be enlarged, do so carefully with a small pair of *clean* scissors. Remember to think about whether your hands are clean, since this nipple will be going into the foal's mouth. Most foals need a relatively large nipple, one that approximates the size of the mare's nipple, so the Playtex brand of baby bottle that has a more human-sized nipple will not be very useful. The classic human baby bottle usually is quite adequate, but another useful alternative is to buy the black rubber sheep's nipple that is available in most feed stores. These nipples fit securely over the rim of most soda pop bottles and make a nice system for bottle feeding a foal. Remember that the bottles must be very clean and free of detergent residues that may cause stomach upset.

BOTTLE FEEDING THE FOAL

If this bottle feeding is only a stepping stone to natural nursing, it is important to give it to the foal in a manner that will not cause him to associate the food source with some entity apart from the mare's udder. To give the bottle to the foal, tease his upper lip gently with the end of the nipple, and if he responds with interest, lure him over to the mare's side in approximately the proper nursing position, hindquarters against the mare's shoulder, head facing her flank. With your valuable assistant at the mare's halter to control the mare's behavior, stand on the side of the mare opposite the foal and reach under her belly to offer the bottle to the foal. A third person may be needed to steady the foal, since he may forget to balance himself when he realizes that milk is available. Do not try to push his head toward the nipple, since this will always be met with resistance and struggle. Instruct your assistant to touch the foal *only* when it is necessary to steady him or to adjust his body position with respect to the mare. Touch his upper lip with the nipple, and when he responds to it, slowly pull the nipple back into approximately the region of the mare's udder to teach him that successful feeding is associated with the mare's udder. Whenever you move the bottle to guide the foal's mouth, move it slowly and do not get too far ahead of him so that he loses his way. Resist the temptation to bring the milk to him—rather, teach him that he must bring himself to the milk. In this way, the transition from baby bottle to mare's udder will not be a difficult one. Be sure that the bottle is tilted so that milk will flow through the nipple. This will reinforce the foal for being in the right location, it will strengthen his sucking reflex and it will prevent him from sucking air into his stomach. As soon as the bottle has been drained, pull the nipple out of his mouth so that he doesn't suck air.

If circumstances dictate that the foal will be raised as an orphan, apart from his dam, a particular location should be chosen for his feeding. In most cases, the feeding location is a

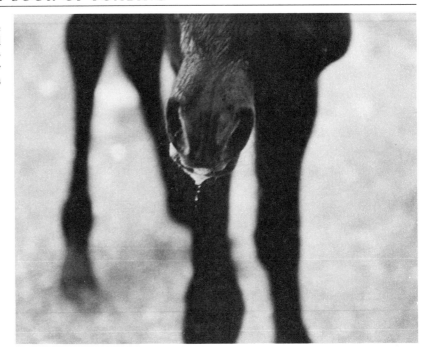

certain corner in the stall, or a certain location near the gate. Whatever you choose as your feeding location, try to keep it consistent—try to feed the foal in the same location every time. Otherwise he will begin to associate feeding with *you* rather than with that location, and every time you enter his stall you'll be "mugged" by the foal. This may seem cute at first, but you may feel differently about it in a few weeks when he outweighs you.

As long as a bottle is being used, remember to keep it tilted so that the foal sucks *milk* into his stomach, not *air*. Remember to give him an adequate quantity of good-quality mare colostrum during his first 12 hours of life, then begin to switch him over to the milk product of your choice. Acceptable substitutes for natural mare's milk include fresh or frozen goat's milk, fresh or frozen mare's milk from another mare, natural nursing from a surrogate mare or any of the commercially prepared mare's milk replacers. Cow's milk must *not* be used, since the content of natural cow's milk differs too much from mare's milk, leaving the foal deficient and often creating fatal scouring (diarrhea). Many of the commercial calf milk replacers are likewise not advised, since their composition often contains levels of vitamin D that are highly toxic to foals. If they aren't supplemented with vitamin D, some of the acidified calf milk replacers can be used successfully and are generally a more economical choice than the products made specifically for foals. Don't be confused, though—an *acceptable* substitute is not necessarily the *ideal* choice, and whenever budget and availability permit, a milk replacer designed specifically for foals should be used.

Section 5.4
Identifying the ''At-Risk'' Foal

During the first hour after birth, the newborn foal should be examined by the foaling attendant and veterinarian to ascertain whether any abnormalities are present. The history of the pregnancy as well as the history of the mare, the stallion and the premises should be considered in order to identify any tendencies, predispositions or increased risks for potential problems. A checklist of things to look for after a routine foaling can be found in Chapter 6 following the summary of the normal equine birthing. In this section, however, we'll take a more detailed look at some specific abnormalities and some conditions and circumstances that place the newborn in the special category of *foal at risk*.

Even when a birthing occurs without problems, the foal appears perfectly normal, and veterinary examination reveals no abnormalities, the foal can harbor problems that are subtle or invisible at first but which can become significant all of a sudden. When the foal is identified ahead of time as an at-risk foal, special precautions can be taken to observe him more closely so that the smallest hint of a problem can be detected and acted upon before the problem gets out of hand. By the same token, certain "abnormalities" are actually "normal" under specific circumstances, and the veterinarian and caretaker will be much less inclined to institute unnecessary treatment when they are better informed about what "abnormal" conditions to tolerate in the newborn foal. In the following pages, then, specific abnormalities (as well as "normal" or "acceptable" abnormalities) are listed with descriptions of what to look for, what to expect and what to do about it.

1. The foal is a dystocia foal

Any foal experiencing a difficult and/or prolonged delivery is at risk of oxygen deprivation (hypoxia) and blood deprivation (ischemia) from spending too much time "in limbo" in the birth canal while his blood supply is slowly and progressively being cut off because the placenta has started separating from the uterus. Both conditions can lead to cellular damage in the brain, and the extent of the damage will depend largely on the degree and duration of the deprivation. In many cases the foal appears to be perfectly normal at first and does not exhibit any signs of brain (cerebral) dysfunction until he is a few hours old. This is because much of the dysfunction occurs as a result of swelling in the brain, and this swelling can be slow to develop if the insult to the tissues was on the lower end of the severity scale. In milder cases, the foal seems normal in all ways except for impaired ability to learn simple tasks such as rising, balancing, walking, suckling and/or nursing.

As a general rule, **when cerebral swelling and cellular damage are minimal, the first thing to go is the suckle reflex**. Even

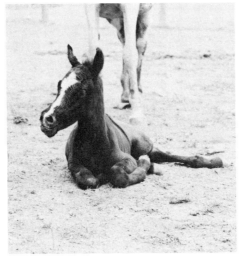

FIGURE 5.08
The normal foal will exhibit a suckle reflex long before actually connecting with a nipple. If there is a mild cerebral problem, his suckle reflex may be temporarily impaired and this behavior will be diminished or absent.

when the foal is more seriously impaired, his recovery does not necessarily require placement in an intensive-care facility as long as his needs are recognized and met. Obviously the more severe his impairment, the more technology will be required in providing appropriate treatment and the lesser are his chances of recovery.

If the foal seems normal in all ways except for a lack of suckle reflex, treatment will consist primarily of measures to provide essential colostrum and nourishment. He may exhibit normal signs of hunger, probing around his dam as though looking for her udder, but there is diminishment or absence of the usual "sucking air" behavior whereby the normal foal sticks out his tongue, wraps it around his upper lip and sucks. In addition to his eventual weakening from lack of nourishment, this abnormal behavior can eventually irritate the mare, since the foal will continue to probe and nudge without giving her any of the gratification of suckling.

PLAN OF ACTION:

a. Milk the mare, check colostrum quality and, if it is of good quality, offer eight ounces to the foal in a baby bottle, using proper technique. If the quality is not good enough, offer banked colostrum from your freezer. If the foal shows no interest in suckling the nipple, squirt 5 cc (1 teaspoon) of light corn syrup into his mouth with a syringe, wait a few seconds, then offer the bottle again. Often this intense sweetness heightens his awareness of his mouth and tongue and gets him suckling. If still no luck, the veterinarian will have to pass a small-gauge (newborn foal size) stomach tube into the foal's stomach and give the 8 ounces of colostrum by gravity feed through a funnel. Let the foal sleep for a half hour after feeding, then gradually get him up (if he doesn't get up on his own) and let him walk around for another half hour (a total of one hour from feeding) before trying to feed again. Try the bottle without the corn syrup first to test for the presence of his suckle reflex. If still no luck, try the corn syrup trick again and give him another bottle of colostrum, or have him tubed again if the suckle reflex is still not present. Keep track of the feeding times and volumes so you'll have a record of how much colostrum he is getting compared to how much he needs (see page 167). In almost all cases, the foal becomes more and more normal after digesting each successive feeding. If the results are less than promising, bear in mind that the newborn foal can tolerate only a small amount of sucrose (the kind of sugar found in corn syrup) before digestive upset results. If this trick is going to work, just a small squirt is all that is usually necessary.

Note that although it is possible to force-feed a foal orally by squirting milk into his mouth with a large syringe, this is not a recommended approach for three reasons: (1) It can lead quite easily to aspiration of milk into the foal's lungs, since the foal will probably struggle against your efforts and may take some of

FIGURE 5.09
The normal foal can right himself to the sternal position without assistance by the time he's about 20 minutes old.

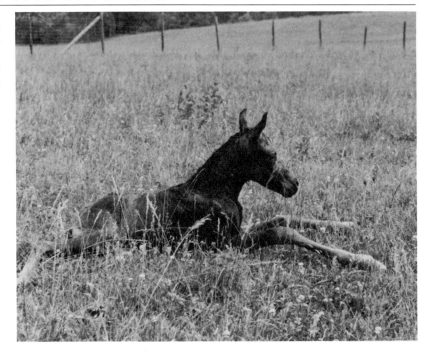

the milk down the "wrong tube" (the trachea), leading inevitably to pneumonia. (2) The entire process of force-feeding is usually met with resistance from the foal, creating a prolonged stressful encounter with every feeding. In many cases, particularly when the foal is hypoxic, stress will lead him to "phase out" by suddenly becoming completely limp. If this happens, just lay him down gently and let him sleep, and while he's sleeping, try to figure out a less stressful way to get him fed. Having him "tubed" may seem stressful to you, but it only lasts a few moments, and then it's over. (3) Force-feeding by syringe is bound to be wasteful, since the foal will do everything he can to keep from swallowing the milk you place in his mouth. The wasted milk that falls on your shoes is not just milk—it's colostrum, which should be handled like liquid gold.

    b. The veterinarian will have to decide whether the use of intravenous medications for treatment of cerebral swelling is warranted. Several agents are appropriate; a current favorite of equine neurologists is medical-grade dimethylsulfoxide (DMSO) diluted appropriately in sterile saline and administered by aseptic technique. In cases of cerebral swelling due to head trauma, I have seen this treatment, given in conjunction with intravenous dexamethasone, produce immediate results that are nothing less than miraculous. Its use in any case, including the compromised neonatal foal, however, must be judicious and with full knowledge of potential side effects. For example, if there is cerebral hemorrhage, the DMSO may prolong clotting time, encouraging the bleeding to continue longer. **For this reason, field use of this treatment should be limited to foals with severe and worsening signs of cerebral swelling, including inability to stand and walk.**

c. The veterinarian will also have to decide whether the foal should be treated with antibiotics, since his condition could be associated with an ongoing infection in the placenta that could have spread to his own system. Furthermore, he is at risk of picking up a *new* infection due to his compromised condition. Some veterinarians will choose to submit blood samples for a blood culture and will prescribe antibiotics only if a specific infectious organism is isolated within 48 hours. Others will choose to start the foal on a regimen of broad-spectrum antibiotics right away on the *assumption* that an infection is present or imminent whether or not it can be identified. There are advantages and disadvantages to both approaches, and arguing the finer points of pharmacology is beyond the scope of this book. If empirical treatment with antibiotics is started, it is essential that the treatment continue for a minimum of six days, even if the foal appears normal before then, since bacteria can develop resistance to antibiotics when given for only a short period.

Other options to include in treatment are intestinal inoculants ("good" bacteria for the intestines), immune system stimulants, and anti-ulcer medications to protect the foal's stomach against ulcers, which are common in the "stressed" foal.

d. Be sure to meet all his "routine" needs, such as tetanus antitoxin, iodine for his navel and an enema.

2. The foal is a "slow" foal

Some foals are slower learners than others, particularly with respect to their ability to learn to nurse from their mothers. If it takes a couple of hours for them to get the hang of it, that's probably still within the range of normalcy. And some foals have a little more trouble learning how to unfold their legs to stand and navigate, particularly when they are very long-legged, and they may be an hour old before they can master the standing position. Again, this is still probably within normal limits, as long as each attempt is more successful than the previous one, and as long as their ability to balance long enough to nurse is perfected before they get weak from hunger. But all foals, regardless of how clumsy they are, should be able to rise to the sternal position from lateral recumbency (i.e., if lying on their side, they should be able to rise up and support themselves on their sternum without help) by the time they're 20 minutes old. This is called the righting reflex. And all foals, regardless of how slow they are, should have a strong and persistent suckle reflex. If your foal is "slow" to the extent that his righting reflex and/or his suckle reflex are deficient, he probably has a degree of cerebral swelling from hypoxia and/or ischemia. This can happen even if his birthing was quick and effortless, because the placenta reserves the right to begin detaching from the uterus, depriving the foal of blood and oxygen, prior to the onset of visible labor, and you may not get any clues that this has taken place.

PLAN OF ACTION:

Follow exactly the same steps as you would in situation #1 above.

3. The mare dripped milk for several hours (or days) prior to delivering

It has long been understood that prepartum dripping of colostrum predisposes the newborn to failure of passive transfer of antibodies due to "wastage" of the valuable colostrum (see Section 5.1). However, the implications of prepartum colostral dripping are actually relevant *much earlier* in the course of the perinatal period, because **premature lactation usually indicates premature separation of the placenta from the uterus.** This places the foal at risk of prelabor hypoxia and ischemia, and he will be born with the cards stacked against his survival. Furthermore, there may be a sinister reason for the placenta to detach prematurely from the uterus, such as inflammation or infection of the placenta (placentitis). This could have grave consequences for the foal, since any infection in the placenta is likely to spread to the foal himself, and you may be presented with a newborn who is ill before he even draws his first breath.

PLAN OF ACTION:

a. If the mare is *at least* 320 days along in the pregnancy (preferably closer to 340 days), if the milk she is dripping is opaque white in color and if the veterinarian finds that her cervix is softened when he or she manually examines it, the best course of action to take with the mare dripping milk is to induce labor and get the foal out of there before he begins to suffer from hypoxia or ischemia. If this is not an option—for example, if the mare does not meet the three criteria for induction of labor, if the veterinarian is not available or is unwilling to induce labor for some reason or if the mare's caretakers allowed her to drip milk unaided because of lack of knowledge, then the only re-course is to be prepared for a hypoxic/ischemic foal and hope for the best. In that case, follow exactly the same steps as you would in situation #1 above.

Note: The three criteria for induction of labor in the equine may be circumvented if deemed appropriate by the veterinarian. A conference between the veterinarian and the mare's owner should take place to discuss the pros and cons of inducing labor in that particular case, and special attention should be focused on the ultimate goals (the realistic ones) regarding outcome in a "worst-case scenario." The most commonly broken rule is the one about the 320 days—remember what was said in Section 1.1 about the arithmetic of equine pregnancy. Many mares foal spon-taneously (and quite normally) prior to Day 320, while others would produce premature foals at Day 340, so the veterinarian is burdened with the responsibility of determining whether or not the foal is developed to a point where his survival is likely if delivered now, and whether he would be better served by risking *prematurity* or by risking *hypoxia/ischemia.*

b. Remember to test the mare's colostrum for quality, since she will only have a finite amount that may have been wasted due to her premature lactation. If the specific gravity of her colostrum indicates that it is less than excellent, provide the foal with the requisite volume of colostrum from your cache of banked colostrum.

4. The pregnant mare has a vaginal discharge

The diagnostic trick here is to determine exactly *what* the discharge consists of and to decide whether the *source* of the discharge is the vagina, the cervix or the uterus. Since the cervix is supposed to be tightly closed during pregnancy, it is unlikely that a discharge would be coming from the uterus (if the pregnancy is intact). If it *is* coming from the uterus, though, the pregnancy is either about to be delivered and/or it is in serious trouble. The *timing* of the vaginal discharge would be important in this case as well, since the fetus is more likely to succumb to *in utero* infection when the exposure to the infection occurs early in his development. If the discharge is determined to be pus (purulent), there is definitely an infection. If it is only mucus, not pus, then there is simply some irritation or inflammation somewhere, probably in the vagina, and as long as the cervix is closed, the pregnancy should be safe. Any previous intervention involving veterinary examination of the vagina (such as a manual or speculum exam of the cervix) will irritate the vagina sufficiently to cause it to secrete mucus, which it will then discharge for the next couple of days. Naturally occurring vaginitis, such as would occur if the conformation of the mare's perineum (the region of the vulva and anus) is faulty and permitting fecal matter to soil the vagina, can produce the same symptoms. So the treatment of the mare and/or the foal will depend quite heavily on the diagnosis attached to the vaginal discharge.

PLAN OF ACTION:

a. If the discharge is determined to be the result of an infection in the uterus or in the vagina, all efforts should be made to determine the identity of the infectious organism. The earlier this is done, the better. Cultures of the discharge must be taken without disturbing the cervix and threatening the safe harbor of the ongoing pregnancy. Care must be taken to interpret the results of the culture intelligently, since even the normal vagina will usually be "dirty" (have positive culture results). For best results, the laboratory report should be submitted to a veterinary clinical pathologist for interpretation—most commercial veterinary laboratories and all universities with veterinary schools have a board-certified clinical pathologist on staff. The laboratory should provide the identity of the organism and a list of antibiotics to which the organism is susceptible. The veterinarian should then prescribe an appropriate antibiotic to be given to the mare prior to foaling and, if necessary, to the foal after he is born. If the infection is only in the vagina, not in the uterus, chances are the foal will not be exposed to it until he is forced through the birth canal during delivery. The veterinarian will have to decide whether that exposure is sufficient to warrant antibiotic treatment of the foal after birth.

b. As soon as possible, examine the placenta for evidence of infection. If it is swollen, discolored, overly heavy or otherwise abnormal, then it is probable that the infection involved the placenta. This means that its ability to provide blood, oxygen and nourishment to the fetus was impaired. In this situation, the foal must be treated as a hypoxic/ischemic foal, and you should follow exactly the same steps as you would in situation #1 above.

c. The veterinarian should also focus on treatment of the mare after foaling, since her future health and productivity may depend on getting the infection in the uterus cleaned up right away. The uterus is extremely vulnerable right after foaling, and any infection allowed to remain there may be absorbed directly into the bloodstream, causing severe blood poisoning (endotoxemia) which can lead to lack of milk (agalactia), founder (laminitis), colic and even death.

5. The mare is aged, has had chronic health problems, is of poor nutritional status, had ventral edema during the latter stages of the pregnancy or has had a uterine biopsy that yielded a Kenney score of 3, indicating that there is considerable scar tissue in the uterus

Remember the chorionic villi, the little "fingers" of the placenta that embed into the uterus to form the Velcro-like attachment? (For a review, see Section 4.2.) These are the ultimate source of the life-giving blood that flows from the mare to the developing fetus during pregnancy. All of the conditions listed above can lead to hypoplasia (retarded development) of the chorionic villi and/or inadequate implantation of those villi into the uterus, both causing a "choking off" of the fetus's lifeline that becomes more and more deadly as he grows larger and in need of in-

191

creased blood supply. In severe cases, the fetus grows and develops as far as he can with the available blood supply, until his blood demand exceeds what the utero-placental unit can provide, and he dies. This is the reason for many of the unexplained late abortions and stillbirths, where necropsy examination of the dead foal yielded no answers as to why he died when he looked so normal. In less severe cases, the foal is, once again, deprived of blood and oxygen, and the effect of this deprivation depends on whether or not he was deprived for a long enough period of time to suffer cellular damage.

Sometimes a problem with the placenta will cause problems long before the foaling process. In the extreme cases, if the flow of blood nutrition from the uterus to the placenta and ultimately to the foal is impaired sufficiently to interfere with normal development of the fetus, he will suffer from a form of growth retardation known as *asymmetrical growth retardation*. This means that although his overall external appearance seems normal in size and proportion, his internal organs are either underdeveloped or have undergone some deterioration. These pregnancies often are prolonged, going way past the average 340 days, because the abnormally developed fetal brain is sending confusing messages to the mare's hormonal system. Most asymmetrically growth-retarded foals are stillborn.

PLAN OF ACTION:

If your mare has one or more of the above conditions, *assume* that her foal is at risk for hypoxia/ischemia and be prepared to follow exactly the same steps as you would in situation #1 above. Unfortunately, mares with less than optimal placental *development or attachment* are more likely to undergo premature *detachment*, leading to further blood/oxygen deprivation for the foal. This creates a horrible dilemma for the veterinarian, since the fetus may suffer from retarded development due to impaired nourishment from the insufficient placenta, meaning that it may take longer for the fetus to develop completely before he is ready to be born. Nevertheless, it may be necessary to induce labor and abbreviate the fetus's time *in utero* because the insufficient placenta is now beginning to detach from the uterus. So the odds of delivering a premature fetus when inducing labor are increased when the mare has one or more of the above conditions, and the veterinarian and mare owner *must* confer about the situation and arrive at a plan of action together.

6. Too many previous foals produced by this mare became sick or died shortly after birth

The truth is, even *one* foal dying is too many. But if this mare exhibits a pattern of producing sickly foals, there may be a problem that could be associated with her colostrum.

PLAN OF ACTION:

a. Approximately two weeks prior to foaling (anytime after Day 300 of the pregnancy), have a blood sample from the mare and from the stallion sent to a special veterinary laboratory for blood-type testing. The laboratory at the University of California at Davis has extensive experience with this particular kind of testing and is at the forefront of recent research developments in uncovering blood incompatibilities. The abnormality (or the *tendency* toward this abnormality) that the lab is looking for is the condition called neonatal isoerythrolysis (NI). In NI, the mare's immune system actually develops antibodies against the red blood cells of the foal, as though those red blood cells were disease-causing germs. It is, in effect, an immune system error. During the first 12 to 24 hours of the foal's life, when his intestinal tract permits absorption of antibodies from the mare's colostrum, he is at risk of absorbing these faulty antibodies, which will actually attack and kill his own red blood cells. This condition is often (usually) fatal.

Usually a foal with NI becomes jaundiced (icteric) as his gums (mucus membranes) and the whites of his eyes (sclerae) turn yellow after the first day or so of life. This is due to an overabundance of pigment in his circulation (from the millions of his red blood cells that have been attacked and killed by the colostral antibodies). The odds are against his survival unless he can be cared for in an intensive-care situation in a hospital setting. The most successful way to treat it is to predict it ahead of time and prevent the foal from drinking the "bad" colostrum.

So: submit the blood samples before foaling, and if the pairing is identified as an at-risk pairing, **be there when the foal is born so that he can be prevented from nursing from his dam** by applying a muzzle, by staying with him constantly for the first 24 hours and by milking the mare out and discarding the colostrum. Provide him with an alternate source of colostrum until he has had the requisite 30 ounces and the 24 hours from birth have passed. Just to be on the safe side, test the mare's milk at 24 hours for specific gravity, and allow the foal to nurse only when the specific gravity has dropped to 1.040 or lower.

b. If the results of the blood tests do not indicate a risk of NI, be especially certain to **be there when the foal is born so that you can test the mare's colostrum for quality by assessing its specific gravity**. Some mares, even when their nutritional status and overall health are excellent and even when they are outstanding producers of milk, produce colostrum that is simply worthless with respect to antibody content. In this case, saving the foal is simply a matter of providing him with good-quality colostrum from a colostrum bank before he nurses from his dam and gets filled up on her worthless colostrum. Unfortunately, getting a foal to take colostrum from a bottle is difficult once he has learned how to nurse from the real thing, so it will be much more convenient to get the banked colostrum into him before he learns to nurse on his own. You will have to milk out the mare every hour so that her milk production will continue after the crucial first 12 hours. This will also help by cutting down on the amount of milk the foal will get if he foils your efforts and manages to sneak a "natural" meal when your back is turned.

Even if the foal has received adequate volumes of excellent-quality colostrum, there is no guarantee that his digestive system is functioning properly and allowing him to *absorb* the antibodies from the colostrum. The only way to know for sure whether he has adequate levels of protective antibodies in his *bloodstream* is to have his blood examined for the specific type of antibody known as IgG. Technology has made great strides in developing an accurate and relatively easy field test for foal IgG, and most veterinarians who specialize in equine medicine will carry a test kit in their mobile units or have one at their home office. The test is based on a process known as radioimmune assay (RIA), and the most common brand of test kit is called the CITE test.

The foal must be at least 18, and preferably 24, hours old in order for him to have absorbed as much as possible of the colostral antibodies he consumed. Ideally his IgG level should be at least 800 mg/dl (milligrams per deciliter). A level of 600 mg/dl is considered acceptable. If the blood tests any lower than 400, the foal is at risk of succumbing to any of the myriad of infectious organisms that live in our environment, and he is a good candidate to receive an intravenous infusion of hyperimmune plasma. Whether or not to subject him to the stress of the infusion process will depend on his current condition, value (emotional, financial or otherwise) and on the results of a serious discussion on the subject between the horse owner and the attending veterinarian. Additionally, no decision should be made on the basis of one blood test. If the blood test indicates that the foal is deficient in IgG, the test should be repeated to be sure that there is no mistake. Hyperimmune plasma is available commercially from many veterinary supply companies and is shipped (and stored) frozen. Alternately, plasma can be harvested from a blood donor horse and administered to the foal as long as the donor is of a compatible blood type. Blood-typing in horses is more complex than in humans and requires access to a commercial or university veterinary laboratory, a luxury not available to most of us. It also requires a certain amount of time, which is also a rare commodity when dealing with a neonatal foal. In a pinch, a stallion or gelding of unrelated breeding (preferably a different breed entirely) can be used as a donor, remembering that there is a small but real possibility of an adverse reaction if the blood is incompatible or impure.

As a general rule, one liter of good-quality plasma administered intravenously to the foal by proper technique will raise his overall IgG level by about 200 units. If the foal is ill, however, he may be using up those antibodies as fast as they are administered, and he may require several liters over a period of a few days. The status of the foal's IgG level should be monitored with repeated CITE tests to determine if additional infusions are necessary.

c. If both (a) and (b) yielded no abnormalities, consider that the foal has a congenital recessive abnormality known as combined immunodeficiency (CID). The diagnosis of CID is one that requires specific laboratory confirmation. It is of paramount importance to make such a diagnosis accurately, since it implicates both mare and sire as carriers for the trait, and the suggestion of this diagnosis, especially when not stated carefully, can elicit a knee-jerk reaction resulting in serious damage to the reputations of the foal's parents. CID is a condition that is most commonly diagnosed in purebred Arabian foals, although it has also been diagnosed in foals of other breeds. It is a hopeless condition, because it prevents the foal from developing antibodies of his own against the myriad of germs he will encounter in his lifetime. Therefore, most foals with CID will live for a short time, while holding onto the apron strings of their mother's colostral antibodies, and then when that passive immunity begins to fade, they become fatally ill.

The best course of action when CID is a factor is to make every effort to get a definitive diagnosis one way or the other—in other words, was it CID or not? "Maybe" is not an acceptable answer, because it points an accusing finger at the sire and dam that may cause irreparable damage to their reputations. If it was CID, then that particular breeding should never be repeated, since it is much more likely to produce another CID foal than if different parents were selected. If a foal becomes ill and dies, and if CID is suspected, definitive diagnosis requires the following:

1. a blood sample taken from the foal **before it nursed or received any colostrum at all.** A foal with CID will have no detectable serum IgM prior to suckling. Almost all normal foals *will* have detectable serum IgM antibodies prior to suckling. If your mare has a history of producing sickly foals, take a sample of blood from this foal right away, before he stands and nurses, and submit it to a veterinary laboratory for IgM analysis.

2. laboratory analysis of the thymus gland. If the foal dies, he should be necropsied and a sample of his thymus gland submitted to a veterinary pathology laboratory for examination under the microscope. Affected foals possess only rudimentary thymic tissue; i.e., the development of the thymus is retarded in foals with CID. If the architecture of the thymus is basically normal, or if it looks like it developed normally but was later damaged, then the foal did not have CID.

7. The foal is overdue (past 340 days), the mare has very little udder development, the mare had access to fescue pasture, the

placenta was abnormally heavy, or the allantois-chorion required manual rupture in order for the water to break

If one or more of the above conditions applies to your mare, there is a possibility of inflammation (placentitis) or swelling (edema) of the placenta. Although exposure to fescue grass pasture or hay is not a prerequisite for placentitis, the "fescue syndrome" can encompass every one of the conditions listed above. The fescue syndrome is associated with the following:

1. Prolonged gestation
2. Thickened placenta
3. Increased incidence of premature separation
4. Inadequate milk supply (agalactia)
5. Weak foals

> Special Note: As a general rule, if the placenta is inflamed and/or infected, it will be abnormally heavy from the excess liquid associated with swelling. The normal placenta weighs approximately 11% of the foal's birthweight (about ten to fifteen pounds).

Whether or not the placentitis is caused by fescue grass, the ramifications are very serious for the foal. An inflamed placenta is less able to provide the developing fetus with blood. In the earlier stages of pregnancy, when the fetus is still relatively small, a decreased overall supply of blood may not be significant. But the bulk of growth in the fetus occurs during the last trimester of pregnancy, and the fetus requires the best possible blood supply to support that growth and to maintain baseline functioning of its enlarging body.

With this in mind, you should begin to suspect placentitis whenever a mare is approaching the late stages of pregnancy (Day 320 or beyond) and still shows no sign of udder development. If no progress is made as the days pass, the probability of placentitis becomes more real, and you are faced with increased odds that the foal will be weakened, critical or dead at birth.

PLAN OF ACTION:

a. If the grass or hay being fed contains fescue, or if you are unsure of the content of the grass or hay, take no further chances. Remove the mare from the pasture and lock her in a drylot or a stall so that the only feed she gets is what you give her. Obtain hay from a known source of excellent quality, certified to be free of fescue. Try also to obtain only untreated hay—i.e., hay that was baled without the use of chemical "conditioners," which some farmers spray on the hay to retard fungal growth, enabling them to bale it before it is properly dried. Since the kind of hay grown and the methods for baling hay are often the same within a particular geographic region, it may be necessary to obtain your hay from an out-of-state supplier. If it's important to you to maximize your chances of a healthy foaling, do not talk yourself out of this added trouble and expense—the importance of "safe hay" cannot be overemphasized. Although most investigators recommend at least 60 days of fescue-free forage for healthy foalings, some researchers of fescue toxicity have found that the ill effects of fescue forage can be reversed in just a couple of days.

b. Make certain that somebody knowledgeable in attending foalings is with the mare at all times—don't leave her alone for a minute, because mares with placentitis often foal with no prior warning. Premature separation of the placenta from the uterus is almost a certainty when the placenta is inflamed or swollen, so the foal is at risk of hypoxia and ischemia, necessitating that you follow exactly the same steps as you would in situation #1 above. Furthermore, when the placenta is swollen, it is tough and more resistant to rupture, so it is more likely that the allantois-chorion will need to be manually ruptured. If nobody is present to do this, the foal is almost certain to die. The amnion is also likely to be swollen, so even if the foal is delivered alive, he may suffocate within an amnion that failed to tear away from his nostrils. And finally, be sure to have at least 30 ounces of good-quality colostrum in your freezer, as well as an ample supply of substitute milk with which to raise your orphan foal, since the mare is likely to have no milk to offer.

c. If the mare has no milk at all and shows no promise of "coming into her milk" in time to feed the foal, the foal will have to be raised on a bottle or pan/bucket of substitute milk. When raising an orphaned foal for the first time, it is best to elicit the aid of someone who has done it before. Be sure to follow the mixing instructions on the package of mare milk replacer (be sure to use *mare* milk replacer, not a milk replacer made for calves unless you're sure it doesn't contain toxic amounts of vitamin D), since digestive upset and constipation or diarrhea can result if the solution is made too concentrated and malnutrition can result if the solution is too diluted. The temperature of the solution should never be too warm, since this denatures the protein in the milk and can lead to foal diarrhea. When using a thermometer, try to adjust the milk temperature to approximately 86° F. If no thermometer is available, it is better to give the milk too cool than too warm.

Whenever possible, the foal should be allowed to live with his mother as a "roommate," even if he is not receiving his milk from her. Unless her attitude is abnormal, she will display normal maternal behavior, including protectiveness, and her teaching and disciplinary abilities will help the foal to grow up with normal social skills, both in terms of dealing with humans and with other horses.

8. The mare has been diagnosed as having a condition called hydroallantois during the last couple of months of pregnancy
The mare with hydroallantois has an abnormally increased volume of fluid within the fetal membranes, up to 50 gallons as opposed to the usual 5 gallons. This is the fluid that ordinarily is expelled when the water breaks. Most investigators agree that hydroallantois occurs as a result of a "coding error" in the cells that comprise the allantoic membrane, such that the cells respond to a deranged set of instructions telling them to secrete too much fluid. It is generally believed to be a condition that is *not* the result of something that happened to the mare during the pregnancy; i.e., it is something that was destined to happen as a result of erroneous information coded into the pregnancy at the moment of conception. It is not, therefore, something that could be predicted or prevented, and the only recourse is to try to deal with it optimally when it happens.

Diagnosis of hydroallantois should be suspected when the size of the pregnant mare's abdomen becomes unusually large. Other possible diagnoses should include twin pregnancy, heart and/or liver disease in the mare, and excessive ventral edema (swelling of the lower portion of the mare's abdominal body wall), which can occur from other causes. Any one of the above possible diagnoses could lead to rupture of the prepubic tendon, a wide straplike musculotendinous structure that helps to support the weight of the mare's abdomen. Ventral edema is not uncommon in late pregnancy, and it does not *always* mean trouble. When the edema is painful, however, as evidenced by a

199

resentful response when the area is touched, the prepubic tendon may be in danger of rupturing.

Hydroallantois is usually distinguished by the fact that the distention of the abdomen occurs suddenly over a relatively short period of time—approximately two weeks—rather than gradually as would be the case with twinning or any of the other diagnoses. The veterinarian can further confirm the diagnosis of hydroallantois by rectal palpation, since the fetus is difficult or impossible to reach by rectal palpation in the mare with hydroallantois, and the position of the uterus is abnormally pushed upward toward the mare's spine.

PLAN OF ACTION:

a. When a definitive diagnosis of hydroallantois has been made, all efforts should be made to assure that the foaling will be attended by the veterinarian. Induction of labor should be considered, since the overstretched uterine and abdominal muscles may be unable to assist significantly in expelling the foal. The veterinarian may elect to create a small puncture hole in the allantois-chorion through the dilated cervix so that the excessive fluid drains out in a slow trickle rather than in a gush, since the rapid removal of this fluid may cause the mare to go into circulatory shock. Preventive measures, such as administration of isotonic and hypertonic intravenous fluids and corticosteroids, should also be considered for the protection of the mare.

b. Hydroallantois should always be considered a condition that places the foal at risk. Realistically, however, regardless of the quality of care, most foals do not survive a hydroallantoic pregnancy, and/or they are severely deformed and must be euthanized. The most common deformity is an abnormally enlarged urinary bladder, which occupies so much space in the foal's abdomen that the other abdominal organs are small and underdeveloped. If the foal is alive, he should be considered at risk of ischemia and hypoxia from placentitis, and you should follow exactly the same steps as you would in situation #1 above.

9. The mare is unvaccinated, there is an epidemic of an equine disease on the premises or in the neighborhood, the foaling

occurred in unsanitary surroundings or on wood shavings, the facility is overcrowded and/or poorly ventilated or the foaling area is continuously reused over and over again for successive foalings without disinfecting it

Any one of the above circumstances leaves the foal at risk of exposure to infectious organisms from which he may be inadequately protected. Added factors, such as inclement weather, can be sufficient stress to the foal's system to push him over into an infectious state.

PLAN OF ACTION:

a. Make certain that the foal receives adequate quantity and quality of colostrum within the crucial time limitation. If his dam is unvaccinated, provide him with colostrum that came from a vaccinated mare. If there is an epidemic in the region, try to provide colostrum from a mare that was exposed to the disease but didn't get it, was vaccinated for it or had the disease and recovered from it. Treat the foal's navel with proper iodine solution every hour for at least 6 hours.

b. Make corrections to the facility as soon as possible. Replace wood shavings with clean straw, or if weather permits, turn mare and foal out into a clean grassy paddock or pasture. If the foaling area is poorly ventilated and smells of ammonia, the foal may be better off standing outside in a rainstorm. Obviously, however, some alternate arrangement should be made, even if it means transporting mare and foal to someone else's facility, since the stress of moving them may not be as severe as the stress of remaining in a filthy environment. Prophylactic administration of antibiotics to the foal is not a substitute for good housekeeping.

10. The foal is premature (according to the arithmetic) or *appears* premature (despite the arithmetic)

If the arithmetic suggests that the foal was born too soon, he is at risk of being a *premature* foal. If he was not born too soon, but he looks like a premature foal, he is a *dysmature* foal. Premature and dysmature foals have one or more of the following characteristics.

1. Small overall size
2. Short, silky haircoats
3. Floppy ears
4. Weak (overextended) ankles (fetlocks)
5. Magenta-colored gums

These foals are usually weak, unable to stand and/or support themselves once they have been lifted to a standing position. Unless there is cerebral swelling, they usually have an intact

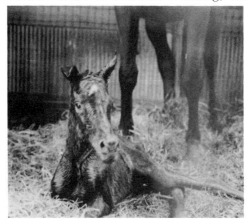

FIGURE 5.10
This full-term foal showed many of the classic characteristics of dysmaturity: small overall size, floppy ears and overall weakness. She was unable to stand until she was approximately a week old.

suckle reflex. The righting reflex is usually intact as well, although they may be too weak to employ it. They are at risk of respiratory dysfunction and/or infection if born prior to completion of pulmonary (lung) development. Dysmature foals are usually the result of a chronic health problem in the dam during pregnancy, and if that chronic health problem is associated with an infectious organism, the dysmature foal may be exhibiting signs of an ongoing infection in his own system.

Retardation of growth in fetuses falls into two categories: symmetrical and asymmetrical. The foal suffering from symmetrical growth retardation is abnormally small all over—all of his parts are equally tiny. This can result from many influences which interfere with growth at the cellular level (mitosis). Mitosis is the process by which one cell divides into two cells, two cells divide into four cells, four into eight, etc. If mitosis is inhibited in any way, the entire foal and all his parts will be growth-retarded. Factors that can cause symmetrical growth retardation include long-term interference with nutrition during fetal development, viral infection in the uterus or placenta during fetal development, abnormalities in the chromosomal or congenital makeup of the fetus and certain medications given to the mare during pregnancy. Phenylbutazone ("bute") is a common offender in this regard; mares with severe chronic lamenesses (such as chronic founder), which must be maintained on high dosages of bute to control their pain, often deliver tiny, growth-retarded, dysmature foals that are weak and definitely at risk.

PLAN OF ACTION:

a. Make certain the foal receives adequate quantity and quality of colostrum. If he is unable to stand and support himself to nurse naturally, you will have to follow the same steps as you would in situation #2 above to assure that he receives the passive immunity and nourishment he so desperately needs to grow and strengthen.

b. The premature and dysmature foal spends more time sleeping than the normal foal. It is more important than ever to be sure the surface he sleeps on is clean, since he will be spending a great deal of time in a position that makes him breathe fumes from the bedding. The bedding should be soft, since his skin is thinner than usual and can be abraded or torn easily. The bedding should provide reasonably good footing, since the foal will make attempts to rise that will be foiled if his feet slip, and delicate tendons can be damaged if he falls "wrong" or "does the splits."

c. If the foal is too weak to do much more than thrash around on the floor, a strict schedule of turning him and re-positioning him should be instituted. If he is allowed to lie on his side for too long, fluid gravitates into the lung lobes closest to the ground and predisposes (or exacerbates) pneumonia. He should be turned over at least every hour around the clock to prevent this accumulation of fluid. Whenever possible, he should be propped up in the sternal position, since this is less damaging to his lungs. Bales of hay make handy cushions for propping the foal. Most foals resent this intrusion, however, and seem to do whatever they can to push themselves away from the bales and lie flat out. Often their movements seem illogical or irrational, and in their thrashing they may abrade or otherwise damage an eye. Bedding may become ground into an eye or into the foal's mouth, and the attendant will need to protect these delicate structures and clean them gently when they become soiled.

d. Normal foals almost always shiver after birth, even if it's 95° F outside, since it still seems chilly after coming out of a 99° F "waterbath." The premature or dysmature foal may have an underdeveloped "thermostat" and be unable to generate enough body heat to keep his bodily functions going properly. The thermostat, which is a sensing system located in the hypothalamus at the base of the brain, stimulates the foal to shiver and create more body heat in order to bring his body temperature up to normal. The premature or dysmature foal may not be able to do this, and the attendant must provide heat lamps or other artificial heating devices to keep the foal's body temperature in the proper range. Be sure to arrange your heating system safely, keeping electric cords out of the mare's reach and keeping hot surfaces away from flammable material such as bedding. Check the foal's rectal temperature often, adjusting the heating system as necessary to maintain the foal's body temperature at approximately 100° to 101.5° F.

In addition to providing auxiliary heat, preventing loss of body heat is another way to help keep the foal warm enough. Makeshift foal blankets can be invaluable, but they should be fitted properly so that they do not restrict the foal's chest when he breathes. Additionally, they should not interfere with his attempts to rise, since he can exhaust himself by struggling to stand when his legs are caught in straps or fabric. By far the best material to use in making a newborn foal blanket is shearling sheepskin, worn with the furry part next to the foal's skin. This creates a soft insulating layer of warmth that will not create undue friction on the thin, delicate skin of the foal, and it will continue to keep the foal warm even when wet.

e. If you can afford it, a natural or synthetic shearling sheepskin makes an excellent "mattress" upon which to lay the foal during his convalescence. By separating the foal from the sharp edges of standard stall bedding, the sturdy but fluffy surface protects the foal's eyes. It is a superior insulator between the foal and the cold hard ground, an important factor even in the heavily bedded stall, since straw will compress with time and lose its insulating properties. Research has shown unequivocally that premature infants of many species, including human babies, puppies, kittens and foals, grow faster, get sick less often and have a higher survival rate when kept on a shearling-like fluffy surface.

Most of the real shearling and the synthetic imitations can generally be machine washed, but this should be investigated thoroughly before making a purchase.

f. If the foal's dam suffered from a chronic health problem of an infectious nature during the pregnancy, the veterinarian will have to decide whether the foal is currently suffering from an infectious condition himself. Appropriate antibiotic therapy should be instituted if this is considered to be a factor.

11. The foal is born during inclement weather

The available facilities will determine how influential the weather is on the stress level of broodmares and their foals. Excessive heat and humidity can be just as treacherous as a polar freeze, and the goal of the attendant should be to minimize the stress to the animals without contributing new stressful factors. Although not directly responsible for infectious conditions, the stress of inclement weather can leave an animal less able to meet the challenge of infectious organisms, creating another at-risk foal.

PLAN OF ACTION:

a. If it is very cold outside, the most important thing to do is to protect the foal from drafts, which can literally suck the heat right out of his body. Most foals are able to create enough body heat to maintain a normal body temperature in subzero weather as long as they are not subjected to a draft. The trick is to eliminate drafts without compromising ventilation, since accumulation of ammonia fumes from urine is just as dangerous as stress from the cold. Extra attention should be given to keeping the stall absolutely clean, since ventilation will be impaired. It is much more important to remove the urine and urine-soaked bedding than the manure.

Alternately, in the colder parts of the country many experienced horsemen practice the deep-litter method of bedding stalls, which actually involves piling fresh bedding on top of the manure rather than removing the manure first. Urine spots are always removed. The base of the deep-litter stall is carefully prepared ahead of time to encourage deep drainage of urine so that ammonia fumes do not accumulate. The thick organic layer of bedding and manure provides insulation from the cold ground and a modicum of extra heat from the slowly composting manure.

b. If the foal shivers constantly, indicating that he is expending too much energy to keep warm, he may not be able to consume enough milk-energy to support normal growth and weight gain. Additional steps should be taken to further prevent heat loss and/or to provide auxiliary heat so that the foal can utilize more of his energy growing and gaining strength.

The safest thing to do with respect to fire hazard is to clothe the foal rather than to install heat lamps or space heaters. A child's sweatshirt with the neck enlarged may be sufficient, but it should be altered so that the foal isn't restricted by it and so that he can't get a foot caught in loose, pendulous folds of fabric. If a sweatshirt is too light-duty for the weather you're experiencing, a polyfill or down-filled vest may be warranted. The synthetics are actually preferable to the down-filled garments, since they continue to insulate even when wet, and since they are more amenable to machine washing and drying. Again, alterations may be needed to eliminate the risk of binding or catching a leg. An excellent garment for cold weather is a baby horse blanket made of shearling sheepskin, worn with the fluffy part against the foal's skin. In severe cold, a combination of garments may be necessary.

If auxiliary heat is used, you should bear in mind that horses are more effectively warmed by radiant heat than by forced-air heat, since the forced-air variety causes a draft which disturbs their winter coats and allows their own body heat to escape. Many types and sizes of heaters are available, and they should be used with the utmost caution and common sense, bearing in mind that barns are full of highly flammable substances and vulnerable living, breathing, trusting animals. Do not make the common mistake of suspending a heat lamp overhead with flammable baler's twine—in all too many instances, the baler's twine ignites and burns through, dropping the hot lamp into the stall and starting a horrific barn fire.

12. The foal has a heart murmur

In most cases, this is one of those "normal abnormalities." A murmur is an ordinarily worrisome sound of abnormal blood leakage through faulty heart valves or rips in the heart muscle, detected when the heart is listened to (ausculted) with a stethoscope. Most foals have some degree of heart murmur, usually of the machinery or systolic variety, immediately after birth. This is the result of some strategically placed openings in the foal's heart, which were necessary for blood circulation while residing *in utero*. When the foal is born, these openings are supposed to heal closed, and this process sometimes takes a little while to complete. In most cases the murmur is gone within the first week of the foal's life. On rare occasions it may persist for a month or two.

PLAN OF ACTION:

Do not make the tragic error of assuming your foal is doomed because of his "heart defect" and have him euthanized. If more foals were examined with a stethoscope, the temporary nature of the murmur would be more widely understood. The plan of action when your foal is discovered to have a murmur is to do nothing. If it persists longer than it should, then it's time to get concerned and consult a veterinary cardiologist.

13. The foal has crooked legs
The description "crooked legs" can mean many things, and the significance of the condition will depend on the diagnosis. The most common abnormalities of foal's legs consist of the following.

1. Contracted tendons
2. Carpal (front "knee") deviations
3. Carpal (front "knee") hypoplasia
4. Windswept foal

The most important approach to crooked legs is to get the problem accurately diagnosed, since the treatment can range from "therapeutic neglect" to physical therapy to surgery by an orthopedic specialist.

Special Note: Just about every foal is born with "crooked legs" (front legs that are slightly valgus [knock-kneed] and slightly toed out). In most cases this is normal, because as the legs grow, which they do in somewhat uneven spurts, the outside surface of the legs finally catches up with the inner surface, bringing the knees out. This naturally turns the toes inward, to a normal straight-ahead position. Normally the legs reach correct alignment by the time the foal is eight to ten months old. Obviously it would be very wrong to "correct" the "crooked" legs of a very young foal with a normal, slight (5 to 7%) knock-kneed/toed-out configuration, because his natural growth that takes place in later months would then create a serious problem in alignment, whereas if they had been left alone, this later growth would have produced straight legs. However, some angular deviations are definitely not normal, depending on their severity, the direction of the angles and the age of the foal. Whether or not to intervene is an important judgment call for the experienced veterinarian.

PLAN OF ACTION:

a. If the foal has contracted tendons, it usually involves the flexor tendons along the backside of his forelimbs. In mild cases the foal is able to rise and stand, but he is a little too far forward on his "tippytoes" because the flexor tendons are too tight. Therapeutic neglect is the best approach in these cases, since the more he uses his legs, the quicker they straighten out. If he occasionally buckles forward onto the front of his fetlocks, you can help him by filing the bottoms of the heels down a bit with a farrier's rasp. Physical therapy can also be helpful. As soon as the foal lies down for a nap, sit down beside him and gently but firmly massage his forelimbs, straightening the legs and rubbing the stretched tendons. Splints and other orthopedic apparati are really not advised, since they tend to interfere with the normal use of the leg (which is the curative influence).

In more severe cases the legs are so tightly held in the flexed (bent) position that the foal is unable to stand up, and if you lift him to the standing position he will buckle and fall. These will most probably require splinting, which the veterinarian will do while the foal is asleep or sedated. The aim of the splint is to hold the leg in the straightened position long enough to stretch the tendons, which is not an easy task on thin, delicate, easily damaged legs. Strategically placed padding and skillfully applied tape is the name of the game. A popular splinting material is a half-round of plumbers' PVC pipe. Some veterinarians will prefer to apply a plaster or acrylic cast to the legs rather than splints, since casts are usually more stable and less likely to slip out of position and create more problems. Casts are usually more expensive initially, and of course their removal necessitates destroying them, so that the tendency is to leave them on longer than needed. The secret to successfully straightening a contracted leg is to leave it splinted or casted only long enough to get the desired results, *no longer*, since the leg is weakened by the appliance and since undesirable side effects (such as pressure sores and impaired circulation) are more likely the longer they are left on. Splints have the advantage here, since they are removed and reapplied often, making it possible to check the progress of the leg and adjust the splint to accommodate changing needs. Removing a cast after it has been on for several days is something of a Pandora's box, since you never know exactly what you'll find on the inside—a beautifully straightened leg or one covered with pressure/friction sores (or worse). An alternate approach when the leg is casted is to remove the cast early by sawing it in half lengthwise, then using the back half as a splint when re-dressing the leg.

In the most severe cases, surgery is prescribed to cut the tendons. This should only be done by an equine orthopedics specialist with an equine anesthesiologist on staff to monitor the delicate foal under anesthesia.

b. There are two processes which can cause the front legs to be crooked at the "knee" (carpus). One is called *valgus* or *varus* deviation, depending upon whether the lower portion of the leg is deviated to the inside or the outside, and it is believed to be the result of uneven growth of the bones. In other words, the medial (inside) surface of the bones is growing faster than the lateral (outside), or vice versa, and the result is a leg that begins to bow in one direction or the other. Although it is mentioned here in this section on abnormalities of the foal seen within the first 12 hours, this is a situation that is usually not recognized until the foal is several days old. However, this condition is difficult to distinguish from another condition that is often present at birth, and for educational and comparative purposes they are presented together here. There are oodles of different recommendations for treatment of the valgus/varus deviation due to uneven growth, and each is as different from the next as night is from day.

I have attended seminars, presented by veterinary orthopedic specialists, where the entire program is devoted to the various surgical procedures advocated to correct the valgus/varus deviations in foals. One procedure involves inserting surgical screws into the faster growing side, wiring the screws together to keep that side from growing, and leaving the apparatus in place until the leg evens out. Placement of the screws is always done under general anesthesia; removal of the screws is either done under general anesthesia or under sedation and local anesthesia.

Another popular surgical approach is called periosteal stripping. The bones are normally "wrapped" in a thin membrane called the periosteum, which contains blood supply and innervation to the bones. When a foal has a carpal deviation, the surgeon strips the periosteum away from the side of the bone that is "growing too fast." It is believed that during the time required for the periosteum to heal, the bone on that side will not grow, while the other side of the bone will continue to grow and will "catch up" with the longer side. The advantage to this procedure over the surgical screw technique is that a second surgery to remove screws is not necessary. Both techniques report reasonably good results.

A third approach is to apply specialized splints to the affected legs. The splints, which are available from veterinary orthopedic specialty supply companies, are designed to apply lateral or medial force on the crooked joint while still allowing it to bend and function normally. They must be applied properly and fitted to the foal's leg according to included instructions in order to avoid pressure sores and improper forces on the leg. Results with this method have also been generally positive.

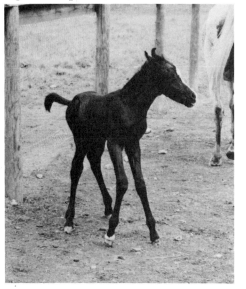

FIGURE 5.11
This mildly windswept foal was able to rise and move about without splints or other leg appliances. Within two weeks his angulations were all within normal limits.

A fourth approach, which was recommended to me by a veterinary orthopedic specialist, is to confine the foal to a small stall "with no appliances" applied to the leg. The little pointy tips on the foal's toes should be rounded with a farrier's rasp so as to encourage a straighter breakover when the foal walks. The rasping may need to be repeated periodically. The length of confinement depends on the legs—some require only 10 days, others require a few weeks before results are seen. The results have been very good, with the deviation resolving in all of thirty affected foals over a two-year test period. The deviation in all of these foals was never more than approximately ten degrees from normal, and most were less than five degrees. The orthopedist cautioned that surgery would be needed in foals with a more severe deviation.

Several foals with equivalent deviation (between five and ten degrees from normal) in my practice were treated with "therapeutic neglect"—their owners failed, for one reason or another, to confine them and trim their toes. To my knowledge, all but one straightened spontaneously without human interference. The one that didn't, which was never presented for diagnosis, is quite crooked as an adult and will probably not be functional as a riding horse.

There is a second, more sinister cause for crooked front legs in foals, called carpal hypoplasia. It is possible that the foal mentioned above with the crooked legs that didn't straighten was a victim of carpal hypoplasia, since this is a condition that requires that the legs be immobilized in plaster or acrylic casts. In carpal hypoplasia, the bony makeup of the carpal bones is incompletely developed, leaving the bones soft and malleable. When the affected newborn foal bears weight on his legs, the soft bones of his carpi become compressed irreversibly, and the longer he is allowed to walk on those legs, the worse the deformity becomes. A diagnostic aid is the fact that carpal hypoplasia is present in affected foals when they are born, whereas in most cases of valgus/varus deviation due to "uneven growth," the deviation is not recognized until the foal is a few days old. The treatment for carpal hypoplasia is to apply casts to the legs to completely immobilize them in rigid extension (no bending is possible with this kind of casting) until the bones harden, which usually takes a few days. The trick is to diagnose the problem before permanent damage is done, and this means that all newborn crooked-legged foals should be examined by a veterinarian immediately in order to determine whether casts are warranted. The presumptive diagnosis is made on the basis of palpation of the legs, and it is confirmed with X rays.

c. The "windswept foal" is usually, but not always, borderline premature. Due to weakness and/or laxity in the tendons, joints and ligaments, his pelvis and hind limbs are deviated variously to one side or the other, giving him the appearance of standing in a strong crosswind. Depending on the severity of the condition, he may or may not have difficulty rising and getting around, which means that he may or may not require assistance with nursing. Once again, treatment for the specific leg problem is usually a matter of doing nothing, as long as the foal is able to get around. In terribly severe cases, support structures have to be custom-made for the foal's specific makeup and weaknesses, but as a rule, any supporting appliances are self-defeating since they tend to foster weakness in limbs that are already pathologically weak. Most orthopedists agree that all but the most severe cases of windswept foals recover spontaneously and grow to be normal, functional adults.

14. The foal is stained with a tacky brown material at birth
This is most likely meconium (foal's first manure), and its presence on the foal suggests that he moved his bowels into the allantoic fluid prior to emerging from the birth canal. The danger here is that he may have inhaled some of this fecal material into his lungs, since the fluids in which he resides circulate in and out of his respiratory tract.

PLAN OF ACTION:

In the ideal situation, the foaling is attended by a well-equipped veterinarian who carries an emergency oxygen setup with suction capabilities. In this instance, the upper respiratory tract is quickly "vacuumed" with the suction to remove any remaining meconium. If this technology is not available, holding the foal upside down, slapping his chest to stimulate coughing and/or cleaning out his nostrils and throat with your fingers may prove fruitful. In any case, he should be watched closely for signs of developing pneumonia. Some veterinarians will opt to start the foal on broad-spectrum antibiotics right away, just in case he did inhale some of the meconium. Others will choose to wait until (if/when) the definitive diagnosis of pneumonia with a specific organism is made.

15. The foal is deformed or abnormally developed
Certain birth defects are congenitally linked, others are merely "accidents" that occurred in fetal development. Unfortunately, the sources of many birth defects are unknown, and there is no consistently sure way of determining whether the deformed foal will grow up to produce others like him or whether he is genetically sound. Some birth defects are so grotesque, debilitating or

otherwise unacceptable that the owner has no trouble deciding to euthanize the foal. Others are less severe and are less clearly defined in terms of their effects on future health, function and productivity. A list of some of the most common birth defects that would require an informed decision regarding treatment plan, future use and/or euthanasia follows.

Common birth defects and deformities:

A. Cleft palate
B. Umbilical hernia
C. Atresia ani
D. Wry nose
E. Dwarfism
F. Microophthalmia
G. Congenital cataracts

H. Hermaphroditism
I. Cerebellar hypoplasia
J. Cerebellar abiotrophy
K. Wobbler syndrome
L. Cryptorchidism
M. Guttural pouch tympany

PLAN OF ACTION:

a. A cleft palate is an abnormal opening along the midline of the roof of the mouth that to varying degrees allows milk to spill into the trachea, leading to aspiration pneumonia. There are several techniques employed to repair a cleft palate; all require major surgery under general anesthesia, and all have less than ideal results. If surgical repair is opted, it must be done as soon as possible so that aspiration pneumonia can be avoided. Alternatively, if a delay in surgical repair is necessary for some reason, the foal can be prevented from nursing and fed with a stomach tube in order to assure that the milk he receives goes into the stomach rather than the respiratory tract. Generally, the outcome of repairing a cleft palate is likely to be disappointing, and in many cases there are other abnormalities present that may or may not be visible. The expense is guaranteed to be substantial. It is generally agreed that this is a congenital defect which can be passed on to progeny, and an animal with a cleft palate should not be considered a future breeding prospect.

b. Repair of umbilical hernias is usually a straightforward procedure that carries few complications, as long as the hernia is not overly large and as long as the integrity of the surrounding tissues is uncompromised. General anesthesia is required, and several surgical techniques are used, ranging from open dissection to closed clamping. There are advantages and disadvantages to both, and the choice of technique should be made according to the characteristics of the specific case. In general, foals with repaired umbilical hernias grow to be normally functional individuals. Unless the umbilical hernia in a particular case can be proven to be an acquired condition, affected individuals should not be considered future breeding prospects, since heritability has been established.

c. Atresia ani is a condition whereby the anus is either sealed closed or not present at all, meaning that the rectum ended before an anus was formed. This anomaly is usually discovered when the caretaker attempts to give an enema.

If surgical correction is elected, it must be done immediately, since the foal will begin to display signs of impaction colic or constipation within minutes to hours after birth. The heritability of this condition is not known, but it is often associated with other concurrent abnormalities. If the accompanying abnormalities are severe, euthanasia is usually elected.

d. Wry nose , also referred to as twisted nose and deviated nasal septum, is a deformity where the foal's muzzle is, to varying degrees, bent to one side. The deviation usually involves the bone and the cartilage of the rostralmost (farthest forward) portion of the upper jaw. Depending on the severity of the deformity, the foal may or may not have difficulty nursing. In the most severe cases, the nasal passages are so crimped that the foal has difficulty breathing.

The heritability of this condition has not been established definitively. Because it occurs more often in horses of the Arabian breed than any other breed, the possibility of a congenital and heritable component is high. It does occur in other breeds, however, and some researchers have suggested that the anomaly can occur as a result of exposure of the pregnant mare to certain environmental factors, such as radiation, drugs or chemicals, certain infections and age-related chromosomal damage. Nevertheless, it does occur significantly more often in female foals than in males, suggesting a sex-linked chromosomal influence.

If surgical correction is opted, the first task is to locate a veterinary surgeon willing to do the surgery. In most cases, surgical correction is done for cosmetic reasons only, since the majority of cases are able to breathe and nurse adequately. The

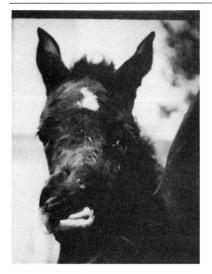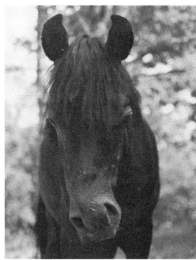

FIGURE 5.12 A,B
If the deformity is not so severe as to interfere with breathing and eating, the wry-nosed foal can usually survive and be somewhat productive. Before surgical repair (a), and after (b).

results are usually a vast improvement on the original appearance of the foal, but they are still a far cry from normal looking.

Some affected foals have difficulty nursing because they can't seem to control their tongues properly, sticking them out of their mouths sideways and lolling them about. Usually a little patient tutoring by the caretaker can get them to take a bottle, manually wrapping the tongue in the proper position around the nipple, until they get the hang of it and transfer their newfound skill to the mare's nipple. If suckling is not possible, wry-nosed foals can be raised as foster babies by providing milk in a bucket or bowl, which they quickly learn to drain. The muzzle is simply dipped into the bowl and the foal does the rest. If the foal is slow to learn, 5 cc of corn syrup squirted into the mouth with a syringe usually gets things rolling.

To date, I am aware of no published or informal reports of wry-nosed foals that produced deformed foals themselves. This is not to suggest, however, that breeding these animals is advocated. Clearly, further work must be done on the underlying cause(s) of this deformity.

e. Dwarf foals are, to some people, irresistibly adorable. Unfortunately, the abnormality is clearly heritable, and dwarfed foals often have other abnormalities that make their lives difficult and short. There is no treatment for the condition, and euthanasia is usually chosen.

215

f. Microophthalmia and congenital cataracts are developmental abnormalities of the eyes that may or may not be heritable. In microophthalmia, the eyes are abnormally small. Detailed ophthalmological examination is mandatory in order to ascertain whether the interior of the eyeballs is normal. Vision tests, which are difficult to do in horses, are also suggested. The most reliable way to test visual function in horses is to construct a maze-type course and observe whether the horse can see obstacles. In congenital cataracts, the lenses of the eyes are abnormally opaque. This is easily observed by examining the eyes with a bright focal light. Surgical removal of the abnormal lenses is possible, but before undergoing the expense it is advised to have the eyes tested to be certain the other internal structures are functioning normally. The heritability of microophthalmia is not clearly defined; congenital cataracts are generally believed to be heritable.

g. Hermaphrodites are individuals with physical parts of males and females concurrently. Since most cases of hermaphroditism are unable to reproduce, it is unlikely that the condition is heritable. As adults, some hermaphrodites can be difficult to handle, since they can exhibit stallionlike behavior whether they are phenotypically male or female. Some cases are sexually and socially aggressive, some are nymphomaniacal and some are sexually and socially passive. If it is desired to keep a hermaphrodite foal for any reason other than to donate it for scientific research, it is advisable to have the animal surgically neutered in order to diminish the possibility of hormonal effects on behavior. Otherwise, the horse may be too unpredictable to be considered safe around people and other animals.

h. Cerebellar hypoplasia and cerebellar abiotrophy are conditions seen most commonly in foals of purebred Arabian breeding. The cerebellum is a portion of the brain that controls motor movement, providing a sense of "where one's legs are" and guiding movement in a smooth and nonspastic manner.

In cerebellar hypoplasia, the cerebellum never develops completely, remaining small and rudimentary. Since it occurs most often in Arabian foals than any other breed, it is believed to be a heritable anomaly. The same condition occurs in cats, however, and in cats the cause has been linked definitively to a viral infection during pregnancy. Nevertheless, in horses most of the evidence thus far points to a congenital component, and breeding of affected individuals is not recommended until further research has been done. Affected horses are treacherous to work around, since their movements are somewhat spastic and unexpected, and using one of these horses for riding would be foolhardy. As a result, most affected individuals are euthanized when the diagnosis is made.

Cerebellar abiotrophy produces exactly the same signs as does cerebellar hypoplasia, but it differs in the sense that affected individuals have normal *development* of the cerebellum, but it deteriorates progressively, to the point of senility, within a few weeks to a few months of age. The diagnostic difference is in the timing—if the foal was displaying signs at birth, he probably had cerebellar hypoplasia. If he seemed normal at birth but gradually became symptomatic by the time he reached the age of two or three weeks, he probably had cerebellar abiotrophy. Currently there is no known treatment for either condition, and the ultimate cause (etiology) continues to elude researchers.

It is likely that there is more than one condition that can lead to cerebellar dysfunction. Some research has led investigators to believe that certain nutritional deficiencies can lead to acquired anomalies of the cerebellum. Dietary deficiencies of copper, zinc and vitamin E have been implicated as possible causes of cerebellar dysfunction. In one study a familial tendency to produce offspring with cerebellar dysfunction associated with vitamin E deficiency was discovered, whereby certain horses of specific family lines were apparently "deficient" in vitamin E when fed a diet that provided *adequate* levels of vitamin E to individuals of *different* family lines. When the affected individuals were *supplemented* with extra vitamin E, their offspring were *not* affected with cerebellar dysfunction. Without the supplemental vitamin E, the offspring they produced displayed signs of cerebellar dysfunction. Once the symptoms of cerebellar dysfunction were present, supplementing the affected individuals did not appear to bring about any improvement. Other horses of separate family lines, residing on the same farm and receiving exactly the same diet, showed no tendency to produce offspring with cerebellar dysfunction, even when not given supplemental vitamin E.

The current plan of action is to watch your foals for signs of

217

poor balance, head tremors, high-stepping rigid movements of the forelimbs and lack of "menace reflex" (the usual avoidance movements a normal foal makes when you pretend that you're going to slap his face). If the problem is diagnosed on your farm, the affected individual(s) should be examined for possible deficiencies and other underlying influences that may point to a correctable environmental factor. A veterinarian who is knowledgeable in the diagnosis of these conditions should be consulted, and referral to a veterinary neurologist may be warranted before electing a course of action. Realistically, most cases end in euthanasia, but all efforts should be made to learn from them in case an underlying cause is identified that could be corrected to prevent further problems.

i. Wobbler syndrome is a diagnosis that is often made erroneously when referring to foals with cerebellar dysfunction. In wobbler syndrome, the cerebellar architecture is normal, but a malformation of the first two cervical vertebrae (vertebrae of the neck) creates pressure on the cervical portion of the spinal cord, resulting in varying degrees of neurological dysfunction. Researchers are not agreed on whether this condition is heritable, since there may be a degree of environmental (including dietary) influence in selected cases.

Signs of wobbler syndrome occasionally are seen in very young foals, but the majority of cases become symptomatic later, during adolescence or early adulthood. Differentiating between wobbler syndrome and cerebellar dysfunction is relatively straightforward, requiring basic knowledge of veterinary neurology and/or a conference with a neurology specialist. Many cases are treated successfully on the surgery table, the important factor being whether any permanent damage has been done to the delicate fibers of the spinal cord prior to surgical alteration of the malformed vertebrae.

j. Cryptorchidism is generally agreed to be a heritable anomaly whereby one (or occasionally both) of a colt's testes fails to descend into the scrotal sac. Both testicles are usually descended into the scrotum at birth, remaining there for approximately two weeks, then returning to a higher position until several months later, when they descend again. It is unclear whether cryptorchids have both testicles descended at birth and then fail to drop one or both of them as yearlings after bringing them up at the age of two weeks, or whether they have one or both testicles retained at birth. Many people simply don't bend over to look for two testes in newborn colts. Diagnosis of cryptorchidism should not be made until the colt is at least a year old, and many investigators claim that you should wait until the colt is two years old, since descent of the testicles is sometimes delayed until then. Fertility is diminished (but not eliminated) when one testicle is retained, since the retained testicle is subjected to body temperature, which is too warm for survival of sperm. Affected individuals should not be used as breeding stallions, since the heritability of the condition has been established.

Castration should be done only when the retained testicle can be located and removed at the same time as the descended testicle, since exploratory efforts to find the retained testicle often depend on knowledge of whether the retained testicle is the right or the left one. If a cryptorchid is gelded improperly (i.e., if the retained testicle is not removed) the horse is likely to exhibit stallionlike behavior, since testosterone hormone production is not affected adversely by the increased temperature associated with being inside the body. Blood testing for the hormone estrone sulfate in geldings suspected of having a retained testicle is a very reliable way of identifying these individuals.

k. Guttural pouch tympany is a condition whereby normal air movement into and out of the guttural pouches is altered. The guttural pouches are two thin-walled sacs in the throatlatch region of the horse, situated at the end of what would be the eustachian tubes in the human. The function of the pouches is not known, but in some horses their dysfunction creates some serious problems.

In guttural pouch tympany, air is allowed to enter the pouches through slitlike openings in the pharynx (back of the throat), but one or both of the valvelike slits malfunctions, preventing the air from escaping. As a result, the pouches begin to fill up and distend, giving the horse's throatlatch a swollen, mumpslike appearance. Unlike mumps, however, the swelling consists entirely of air.

In addition to spoiling the cosmetic appearance of the horse, the air-filled guttural pouches can impinge upon the lar-

FIGURE 5.13 A,B
Foals with guttural pouch tympany, usually fillies, exhibit puffiness in the throatlatch region (one or both sides) and may or may not experience breathing difficulties as a result of the pressure on the larynx.

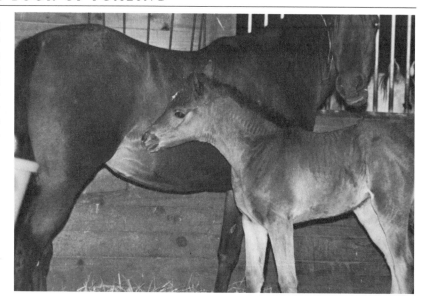

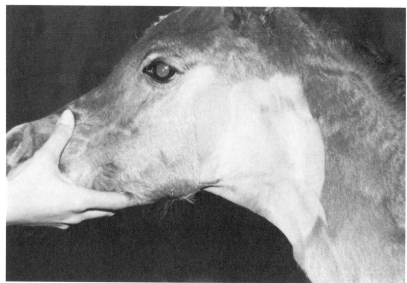

ynx and arytenoid cartilages of the throat, creating breathing difficulties ranging from an audible "snore" to frank suffocation.

16. The foal is dripping urine from his navel

Prior to birth, the foal normally passes urine through a portion of the umbilical cord called the urachus. After birth, the urachus is supposed to seal closed and the foal should urinate through the urethra in the penis (in colts) or the vagina (in fillies). Occasionally the urachus remains open (patent), allowing a variable drip or stream of urine to pass through when the bladder is full or simultaneously while the foal is urinating through the urethra.

If left unchecked, a patent urachus could lead to a number of more serious conditions, including omphalitis (inflammation and/or infection of the umbilical cord stump) and septicemia (an infectious form of "blood poisoning"). Many cases of patent urachus respond favorably to local treatment; other cases fail to respond and require surgical repair. The most rational plan of action is to treat the patent urachus "conservatively" at first.

PLAN OF ACTION:

The treatment for patent urachus is a gentle attempt to irritate the navel just enough to cause it to seal closed. This is usually accomplished by repeatedly dousing the navel in tamed iodine solution or tincture of iodine. The "strong" iodine solution, which is a 7% solution used for hoof thrush and sole abscesses, should be avoided for treatment of a foal's navel, since it can burn the skin and cause ulcerations that may require surgical repair. Instead, use an iodine-based surgical solution such as Betadine or Povidine, being careful to choose the *solution*, not the *scrub* (the scrub forms a lather). If the navel still drips urine after a day or two of treating it every couple of hours, the veterinarian may choose to cauterize it with silver nitrate or with a battery-powered electrocautery unit. In severe or refractory cases, surgery is the only option.

17. The foal's hooves seem incompletely formed

Many people with little or no experience in foaling attendance are unfamiliar with the appearance of the newborn foal's hooves. As a protective measure for the mare's uterus, the tips of the foal's hooves are "capped" with a fleshy material (called "golden slippers")

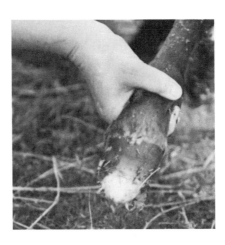

FIGURE 5.14
The protective "golden slippers" worn by all newborn foals are quickly shredded and worn off as they attempt to stand.

221

that makes them softer and less apt to poke through the mare's tissues. The consistency of this material is much like that of raw fish—firm yet somewhat rubbery. After only one or two attempts to stand up, the foal will have succeeded in shredding and abrading the material away from the harder horn of his hooves, thereby making his hooves look normal.

18. There was a piece of liver on the ground after the foal was born—did it belong to the foal?

Now don't laugh, all you experienced horsemen. You'd be amazed at how frightening it is to a concerned owner when it looks like somebody forgot to put the foal's liver inside his abdomen. The topic of discussion here, obviously, is the elusive structure called the hippomanes. The hippomanes is a tan to dark brown–colored mass of tissue, having a consistency much like cooked calves' liver, and usually about the size of a small child's hand. This structure apparently resides within the allantoic fluid and often slips out with the fluid when the water breaks during labor. There are several hypotheses regarding its origin, including the most common contention that it is a conglomeration of the endometrial cups, temporary glandular structures that are necessary for maintenance of the pregnancy during its earlier stages. As the pregnancy advances in development, the endometrial cups are eventually no longer needed, and they are shed from the uteroplacental unit. Each "cup" is about the size of the tip of your thumb and is beige to tan in color during its functional lifetime. It is logical that the discarded cups should coalesce to form a single mass, and as the mass becomes smashed between the developing foal and the mare's uterine wall, it takes on its typical liver-pancake appearance.

19. The newborn foal is breathing very rapidly

Although all vital signs should be evaluated formally by an experienced equine veterinarian, the respiratory rate in normal foals is always high at first. After the first half hour or so of life, it should have stabilized to around 20 to 40 breaths per minute. Additionally, newborn foals are periodic breathers, meaning that their respiratory rate may fluctuate quite a bit as their homeostatic mechanisms come into full function. In premature and dysmature foals, the inconsistency of the respiratory rate may be exaggerated, and this should be taken into account when evaluating for pulmonary (lung) disease. Persistently elevated respiratory rates may also indicate rib injuries.

20. The newborn foal's heart rate is very rapid

Again, all vital signs should be evaluated by a veterinarian, but the heart rate is typically around 130 beats per minute during the first hour of life in a newborn foal. After the first hour, it should drop to less than 120 and usually hovers around 80 to 100 beats per minute. Remember that a heart murmur is usually a "normal abnormality."

21. The foal has an abnormal growth or "tumor"

The differentiation and migration of cells during development of an embryo or fetus are complex and wondrous processes. Every time a completely normal individual is born, we should all marvel over the fact that no apparent mistakes were made during development, because the opportunities for errors are too numerous to fathom. Once in a while, a cell or bundle of cells "gets lost" on its way to its appointed destination, and the result is the growth of a particular type of tissue in a place where you wouldn't ordinarily expect to see that kind of tissue.

In some instances, cells that were assigned

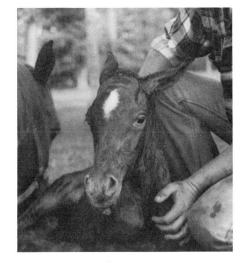

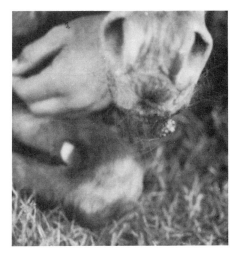

FIGURE 5.15 A,B
An abnormal cluster of epithelial cells on this filly's face was conveniently situated at the end of a slender stalk on her upper lip. Removal was a simple matter of crushing the stalk with forceps and snipping it off.

the task of developing into teeth are detoured, most commonly to the area behind the foal's ear, and the result is a lump under the skin called a dentigerous cyst, which, when surgically opened, is found to contain one or more teeth.

Despite the fact that these particular tooth-developing cells never arrived at their proper destination, most foals with this abnormality are not lacking any of their usual complement of teeth in their mouths, and no other abnormalities are likely to accompany the discovery of the tooth-bearing lump.

Wayfaring dental tissue has been discovered elsewhere in the body as well, including within the structure of internal organs. Ocular tissue (eyeballs, whole or part), hair, fat cells and other normal body tissues have been found in abnormal locations, and besides being interesting to talk about, the fact that they ended up in the wrong place usually has little or no effect on the individual's overall health unless the function of the host tissue is somehow impaired by the abnormal tissue's presence.

The occurrence of this rather benign type of deformity appears to be random, and there are no known reports of genetic or hereditary predisposition to it.

PLAN OF ACTION:

Unless the presence of the abnormal tissue is interfering with normal function of its host tissue, surgical removal is an option that is chosen only if cosmetic improvement is desired. The location of the abnormal tissue may make surgical removal difficult without undue risk to the animal's overall health, such as, for example, when the "tumor" is intertwined around major blood vessels, nerves or ducts. A conference with the surgeon should be sought before deciding whether or not to choose this route. In many cases, the abnormal tissue is located quite superficially on the skin, and it may even be suspended on a "stalk" (pedunculated). In these cases, removal may be as simple as the judicious application of a rubber band. Consultation with a veterinary surgeon should always be included in the decision-making process.

22. The mare has an especially large, swollen area under her

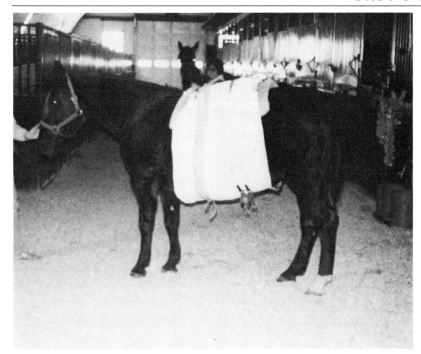

FIGURE 5.16
This Quarter Horse mare's twin pregnancy threatened to rupture her prepubic tendon due to the excessive weight on her belly. A makeshift belly support helped to transmit some of the weight to her backbone and prevented the rupture. Notice the thick padding over her spine to protect against pressure sores. Both twins were successfully delivered vaginally; one survived.

belly, and it seems to be getting larger and larger as the pregnancy progresses

Ventral edema, or swelling of the lower portion of the mare's belly, is not uncommon during the latter stages of pregnancy, particularly in older mares. When the edema becomes excessive, however, and appears to be growing, the mare may be at risk for a condition called ruptured prepubic tendon.

The prepubic tendon is a broad, flat, straplike structure that attaches the lower muscles of the abdomen into the pelvic area, and one of its primary functions is to serve as a support for the heavy abdomen of the mare. This is especially important when the abdominal contents become increasingly heavy, as when a mare is carrying a near-term fetus in her uterus. The prepubic tendon is stretched to (and perhaps beyond) its limits in certain pregnancies, especially when the fetus is abnormally large and heavy, when the mare's overall muscle tone is poor or when the pregnancy consists of twins. The gradual tearing of the tendon's "fabric" leads to increased swelling of the mare's ventral abdomen, and the thickening tissues give her an increasingly distorted, swollen profile.

225

FIGURE 5.17
This mare was less fortunate. The prepubic tendon ruptured, leaving her belly with virtually no support for the weight of her abdominal contents. The foal was successfully delivered vaginally, but the mare was humanely destroyed soon after.

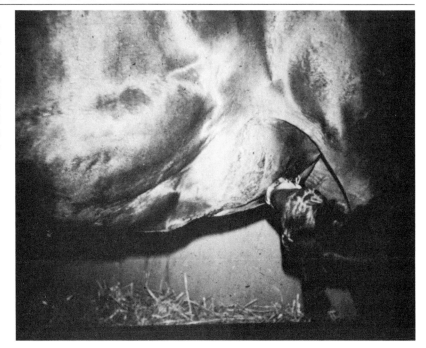

If the prepubic tendon actually ruptures, the mare is basically ruined and is unlikely to survive. Surgical repair of a ruptured prepubic tendon has not been reported to be successful and is rarely (if ever) attempted. The odds are against successfully retrieving the foal from the uterus, since the mare will be unable to provide any significant muscular assistance to the delivery, and cesarean section should be considered.

PLAN OF ACTION:

If the pregnancy is not far enough along for the foal to be adequately developed, steps must be taken to support the mare's stretching and groaning abdomen and prevent prepubic tendon rupture. Administration of furosemide (Lasix), a diuretic drug used to reduce swelling, is not indicated here, since the swelling is merely a symptom of a more serious underlying problem, and the furosemide will only serve to dehydrate the mare.

Effort should be made to stimulate the circulation to the abdominal muscles without contributing any further strain to the area. Exercise that would "bounce" the abdominal contents

226

is obviously the last thing the mare needs, so the next best option would be hydrotherapy—whirlpool therapy. Walking the mare into a warm whirlpool bath up to her belly would be ideal, but most stables are not equipped for such a luxury. A viable alternative is to hose the area with a bracing spray of water for ten minutes at a time, the idea being to stimulate without irritation. This same treatment would also be appreciated by the mare's lower limbs, since they are likely to be swollen as well. Exercise should be limited to walking in-hand.

An abdominal support apparatus can be fashioned with a variety of materials. Care should be taken to provide support without causing harm, such as would occur if the "girdle" were to constrict, pinch, bind or cause friction sores. If possible, a commercially made equine sling should be used, with the sling suspended from the ceiling with just enough tension to lift slightly on the mare's belly but allowing the bulk of her weight to continue to be borne by her own legs. Lacking such sophisticated equipment, a viable alternative is to apply a handmade girdle, using a stiff fabric such as canvas, and padding the mare's spine with a thick-pile saddle pad in order to distribute the weight evenly.

Assistance at the foaling is absolutely mandatory, since the mare will be less effective in her contractions, and since the possibility of twins exists.

CHAPTER 6

QUICK REFERENCE GUIDE

Now that you have read through the entire foaling process, including all the horror stories of things that could happen if something goes wrong, you should have a healthy understanding of why the informed foaling attendant does the things he or she does. Without a deeper understanding about what is happening inside the birthing process, the procedures involved in active foaling attendance may seem too invasive, too "busy-bodyish." Now that you know better, you will never approach the foaling barn in the same manner again.

The following section is a quick reference guide for the normal foaling. The checklist-style format is used so that the foaling attendant can review the order of natural processes and interventive duties at a moment's notice if a memory lapse occurs during the height of the action.

Section 6.1
Being There, Being Prepared

Make up a daily data sheet for each mare past 300 days of gestation. A sample data sheet containing examples of entries, as well as a blank that can be enlarged and photocopied for your use, follow this section. Twice a day, *every* day, formal observations should be made without fail and recorded on the data sheet. Post the sheet in a safe but visible place, along with a pen or pencil for adding notations. At the end of every day, review the recorded data to see if you missed any patterns that could signal the beginning of important changes in the mare's bodily functions.

The data sheet serves two very important functions. First, it gives you a regimented routine of observations to make every day. Second, recording those observations helps to make them stick in your mind and gives you an overview of the direction of a particular mare's progress. Furthermore, any questions the veterinarian may have about the mare's current status can be answered at a glance, and if a conference is required to decide on a course of action (e.g., to induce labor), all the critical data can be found at once.

Well ahead of the expected due date, review the supplies list and take steps to acquire any items missing from your foaling kit. Be sure to have 30 ounces of good-quality colostrum, frozen in 4- to 6-ounce aliquots, in your freezer or someplace where you can get it if you need it, even if you need it in the middle of the night. If you don't use your colostrum, let it be known that it's available for somebody else, and try to replace it with fresh stock for next year.

Anticipate and take care of any deficiencies in your facilities, such as loose boards, exposed nails, uneven stall floors, etc. Reevaluate hay racks, grain feeders and water bucket hooks from the foal's point of view and make any necessary changes to protect delicate (and initially clumsy) baby parts against accidental collision with these objects.

Disinfect the designated foaling area with a safe, broad-spectrum disinfectant such as chlorhexidine (Nolvasan), follow-

PREFOALING DATA, MARE: *Moondance*

DATE	gest. day	8am RT	5pm RT	skin temp	udder sz/tens	nipples	milk
3-1-90	300	98.7	99.3	cool	empty, soft	—	—
3-2	301	98.7	99.4	"	"	—	—
3-3	302	98.6	99.4	"	"	—	—
3-4	303	98.7	99.3	"	"	—	—
3-5	304	98.9	99.4	"	"	—	—
3-6	305	99.0	99.5	"	"	—	—
3-7	306	98.8	99.3	"	"	—	—
3-8	307	98.8	99.3	"	"	—	—
3-9	308	98.7	99.4	warm	"	—	—
3-10	309	98.8	99.4	warm		—	—
3-11	310	99.0	99.4	cool	beginning to fill	—	clear water
3-12	311	98.8	99.5	"	spongey	—	clear water
3-13	312	98.8	99.3	"	spongey	—	clear water
3-14	313	98.7	99.3	warm	about 1/4 full	empty	clear water
3-15	314	98.7	99.3	warm	spongey	empty	"
3-16	315	98.9	99.4	"	spongey	empty	"
3-17	316	98.8	99.5	"	about 1 full	empty	"
3-18	317	98.8	99.5	"	about 1/2 full	empty	"
3-19	318	99.0	99.5	"	half full	empty	clear water
3-20	319	99.0	99.5	cool	spongey	empty	yellow water
3-21	320	98.7	99.3	warm	half full + hard	small	yellow water
3-22	321	98.8	99.3	"	3/4 full + hard	small	yellow water
3-23	322	98.8	99.3	"	full + tense	small	yellow water
3-24	323	98.7	99.4	"	full + tight	bigger	yellow water
3-25	324	98.7	99.4	"	full + tight	bigger	yellow sticky
3-26	325	98.7	99.3	"	full + tight	full	honey
3-27	326	98.6	98.7	"	full + tight	full	skim milk
3-28	327	98.6	99.2	"	full, tight	full	opaque white

KEY TO COLUMN HEADINGS:

GEST. DAY: Gestation (pregnancy) day

RT: Rectal temperature

SKIN TEMP: Lay your hand on her shoulder to see if she is hot or beginning to break a sweat.

UDDER SZ/TENS: The udder increases in size and tension incrementally. Assess daily progress.

NIPPLES: The udder may be full and tense for several days before the nipples begin to enlarge and fill.

MILK: Assess its color, consistency, and note how much effort is required to express it—does flow freely, or do you have to work at it before any milk comes out?

PREFOALING DATA, MARE: *Moondance, p. 2*

body shape	croup	vulva	mucosa color	app/att	sclerae	comments
wide	flat	short	pale pink	normal	N	—
wide	,,	short	—	normal	N	—
"	"	short	pale pink	"	N	—
"	"	"	"	"	N	—
"	sunken	"	"	grouchy	N	—
"	"	"	"	normal	N	—
"	"	"	"	"	N	—
"	"	"	darker pink	"	N	—
"	"	"	pale pink	"	N	—
"	"	"	pale pink	"	N	—
baby dropped ,, "	"	"	"	"	N	—
"	"	longer	"	"	N	—
"	"	longer	"	"	N	—
"	"	"	darker pink	"	N	—
"	"	"	darker pink	"	N	—
"	"	"	pale pink	"	N	—
"	"	"	pale pink	grouchy	N	—
"	"	"	"	grouchy	N	—
"	"	"	"	"	N	—
"	"	"	"	"	N	—
"	"	long	"	"	N	—
"	"	long	"	"	N	—
"	"	long	"	normal	N	—
"	"	long	"	normal	N	—
"	"	long	"	sweet	N	—
"	"	long	"	sweet	N	a little ventral edema
"	"	long	darker pink	sweet	N	"
"	"	long	darker pink	off feed	bloodshot	dripping milk, cowpie-like manure

KEY TO COLUMN HEADINGS:

BODY SHAPE: Silhouette changes to signal when the baby has "dropped"

CROUP: Muscles relax, permitting a hollow in croup region

VULVA: Elongates when relaxed

MUCOSA COLOR: Mucous membranes inside vulva may deepen in pink color as foaling time nears

APP/ATT: Appetite may decrease, attitude may change as foaling time nears

SCLERAE: The "whites" of the eyes (the sclerae) may become injected ("bloodshot")

COMMENTS: Anything interesting or unusual

PREFOALING DATA, MARE:_____

DATE	gest. day	8am RT	5pm RT	skin temp	udder sz/tens	nipples	milk

KEY TO COLUMN HEADINGS:

GEST. DAY: Gestation (pregnancy) day

RT: Rectal temperature

SKIN TEMP: Lay your hand on her shoulder to see if she is hot or beginning to break a sweat.

UDDER SZ/TENS: The udder increases in size and tension incrementally. Assess daily progress.

NIPPLES: The udder may be full and tense for several days before the nipples begin to enlarge and fill.

MILK: Assess its color, consistency, and note how much effort is required to express it—does it flow freely, or do you have to work at it before any milk comes out?

PREFOALING DATA, MARE:_____

body shape	croup	vulva	mucosa color	app/att	sclerae	comments

KEY TO COLUMN HEADINGS:

BODY SHAPE: Silhouette changes to signal when the baby has "dropped"

CROUP: Muscles relax, permitting a hollow in croup region

VULVA: Elongates when relaxed

MUCOSA COLOR: Mucous membranes inside vulva may deepen in pink color as foaling time nears

APP/ATT: Appetite may decrease, attitude may change as foaling time nears

SCLERAE: the "whites" of the eyes (the sclerae) may become injected ("bloodshot")

COMMENTS: Anything interesting or unusual

ing the mixing instructions on the bottle. Whenever possible, leave the foaling stall empty for a week or more before the foaling. Have an alternate foaling area chosen and ready in case circumstances dictate that your first location is suddenly not available or suitable.

Have enough clean, fresh straw (not wood sawdust or shavings!) set aside to keep the foaling area freshly bedded for at least a week, just in case the weather dictates that the mare and her newborn will have to be confined indoors for a period of time.

Have your living quarters set up ahead of time. You may be spending several nights in the barn, so make your setup as comfortable and inviting as possible. If you will be using any electronic devices such as closed-circuit TV or foaling alarms, have them examined in advance to be sure they're working reliably—if they need replacement parts, such as battery packs, tubes or whatever, they may have to be ordered and may not be readily available for immediate shipment.

Have emergency telephone numbers, driver's license, gas money and emergency horse transportation within reach in case a problem should develop. If using your own truck and trailer, be sure the lights and electric brakes work properly, and check the tires (all of them) every day. Have tools in the trailer that can be used to remove the center divider if necessary, and lubricate any joints that may be rusted or otherwise reluctant to slide the way they should.

Section 6.2
Supplies Checklist

Note: *Some of the following are items that should be available on every breeding farm; others are veterinary equipment that should be accessible by the attending veterinarian.*

RESTRAINT ITEMS

General: halter, lead rope, chain shank, twitch

Veterinary: sedatives, general and local anesthetics, analgesics

OBSTETRICAL ITEMS

General: 2 clean buckets, clean warm water, cool water

Tail wraps, baler's twine

Roll cotton, Ivory liquid soap (not detergent)

Sterile individually wrapped plastic shoulder-length gloves

Sterile nonspermicidal lubricating jelly

At least 1 gallon obstetrical lube (OK for vagina and uterus)

Clean bandage scissors

Veterinary: clean large-bore stomach tube

Clean cold-sterilized stomach pump

At least 2 gallons obstetrical lube (OK for vagina and uterus)

Dystocia pack including cable-type hog snare, fetotomy knife and gigli wire

Emergency oxygen setup with suction

Sterile and nonsterile OB sleeves

FIRST AID ITEMS

General and Veterinary: Sterile saline solution (for irrigations)

Clean soft terrycloth towels

Clean soft terrycloth washcloths

Clean lightweight cotton bedsheet

BABY ITEMS

General and Veterinary: Fleet enemas

Tincture of iodine and/or surgical iodine solution (tamed)

Clean cotton twine or string: 12-inch and 36-inch pieces

Emergency colostrum supply, 30 ounces

Clinical refractometer (if vet doesn't have one)

Sterile 8-ounce baby bottle with large nipple

Clean 4-cup plastic kitchen measuring cup with handle

Corn syrup

MARE AFTERCARE ITEMS:
Ivermectin dewormer paste
Bran mash

UTILITY ITEMS:
Flashlight with extra batteries
Bucket with weighted cover for afterbirth
Heavy-duty garbage bags

Section 6.3
Stage I Checklist

• The cervix is softening, allowing the pressure of the pregnancy to press through it, gradually opening it.
• The foal is still upside down at this stage, or the mare's uterus may have just begun to rotate him over to one side. His head and forelimbs should be extended into the pelvis as she rotates him.
• The dilating cervix is associated with release of prostaglandin, which causes the mare general discomfort. Her skin feels warm, you may actually see steam rising from her body and she may break into a sweat. She frequently passes small manure piles, increasingly moist. She may lie down and get up repeatedly, may even roll abruptly onto her back to help the foal rotate in preparation for expulsive contractions. The mare is *not* having expulsive contractions yet.
• The outermost layer of the placenta, the allantois-chorion, is being stretched to its limit as the pregnancy protrudes through the ever-widening opening in the cervix.
• Soon the allantois-chorion will tear ("breaking the water"), so you should be getting ready to check for foal position. You will need to do this as soon as the water breaks, marking the beginning of Stage II. While you wait, try to get the mare's tail wrapped, get the bucket of warm water and put ten or fifteen wads of cotton in it, get the Ivory soap and the baler's twine to

tie her tail, and have your lube, sterile wrapped glove, scissors, string and iodine in your pocket.

Section 6.4
Stage II Checklist

• As soon as the water breaks, wrap the mare's tail, tie it gently off to the right side with baler's twine, wash and rinse her vulva with clean cotton and Ivory soap.

• Put on your sterile glove carefully (don't contaminate it), apply sterile lube generously, slip your hand gently into the vagina and check to be sure there is one muzzle and two fore-limbs.

• Withdraw your hand and back off. The white amnion should be visible at the lips of the vulva; you may be able to see the foal's hoof through the amnion.

• Most mares can push the foal out without help. Labor should begin within 5 minutes from when the water broke. If the mare is slow to begin contractions, a little tug or push on the foal's legs should get things going. On average, it takes about 10 minutes to push him out once she really starts working at it.

• As soon as his muzzle shows, rip the amnion away from it and strip out his nostrils of any foreign material so he can breathe unimpeded.

• Remember the arc-like pathway the foal must follow: he must come up into the pelvis, straight along the pelvis, then down to exit. If it is necessary to pull, visualize where he is within the pelvis and direct your pull accordingly.

• The foal is out. Usually his hind limbs remain in the mare's vagina. Unless he is moving the legs around a lot, leave them in the vagina, since most mares tend to stay quiet longer this way. *(Technically Stage II is over now, but let's get a few more things done before we move on)*

• Check the time. It's preferable (but not mandatory) for the umbilical cord to remain intact for 10 minutes after birth. It will break as soon as the mare gets up, so try not to disturb her.

• Don't wipe the foal off—he's supposed to be wet, and much of the bonding process between foal and dam depends upon the odor of the liquid on his coat.

• Support the foal's tummy with your hand to prevent acquired umbilical herniation. Don't pinch the umbilical cord, in case blood is still flowing through it.

• If the tetanus shot is handy, go ahead and give it to the foal now. Otherwise, it can wait until later, but be sure it's given within an hour or so of the foal's birth.

• Check the foal for meconium stains.

• If you aren't on level ground, try to situate the foal so he can support himself on his sternum or, if he's still too weak, have his head lower than the rest of him so the fluid in his lungs can drain out.

• Be ready with your tincture of iodine or tamed iodine solution and your string (the 12-inch piece). When the mare stands up, concentrate on supporting the foal's tummy against the tension. As soon as the umbilical cord breaks, lean over and look at the stump on the foal's abdomen—is it bleeding? If so, tie it off quickly before he loses much blood. Otherwise, just give it a good soaking with the iodine.

• Note the time.

• Tie up the placenta so the mare doesn't step on it and tear it. If the purple part is sticking out of her vulva, incorporate it in the tie. If not, don't worry about it.

• Back off and let them bond. Remain in the shadows where you can watch, but don't interfere.

Section 6.5
Stage III Checklist

• Keep the lights, the distractions and the noise low. The after-birth will come out a lot faster if the mare lies down to work on it.

• The foal makes several failed attempts to stand and usually succeeds within an hour of birth. Unless the mare is very nervous about your presence, you can give the enema now (and the tetanus shot, if not already done). Give the foal a quick examination for defects such as:

> Atresia ani ("dead-end anus")
> Cleft palate
> Umbilical, scrotal or abdominal hernia
> Congenital cataracts
> Microophthalmia (abnormally small eyes)
> Corneal ulcers (sores or scars on the corneas)
> Uveitis (tightly contracted pupils)
> Petechiae (little pinpoint hemorrhages) on the gums
> Guttural pouch tympany (puffiness in throatlatch)

• All foals are clumsy at first, and some appear to be blind for up to an hour after birth, running into walls and such. This should be temporary unless there's an underlying problem.

• The foal should begin to pass meconium within 15 minutes of giving the enema. He will pass several piles before he's finished.

• He should begin to exhibit a suckle reflex, sticking out his very pink tongue and sucking his upper lip with it. It will probably be at least another hour before he actually nurses from his mother. Meanwhile, he'll suck air, walls, fenceboards and anything else that stands in his way.

• On average, the mare should pass the afterbirth within an hour or two of foaling if the distractions are held at a minimum.

• If the mare and foal appear to be well bonded, remove the afterbirth from the foaling area for examination. If the mare is still unsure of the foal, leave the afterbirth in the foaling area for a little while longer. If she shows suspiciously aggressive behavior toward the foal, lay the afterbirth (or a part of it) over him. It is usually not advised to wipe the foal off with a towel when he's born, since this can remove much of the smell that identifies him as belonging to the mare. The afterbirth may reinforce that smell.

• Once removed from the foaling area, lay the afterbirth out in the same configuration it was in while inside the mare and examine it for missing parts, abnormal color or texture, and thickness. It should weigh from 9 to 12 percent of the foal's body weight, an average of 10 to 15 pounds. If someone wants to examine it again later, submerge it in a bucket of cool water with a weighted cover to discourage flies and critters. Otherwise, dispose of it responsibly.

• Give the mare a nice warm bran mash and some fresh (but *not* ice-cold) water to drink. While she's munching on the mash, take a small sample of her colostrum and check its specific gravity. Ideally it should be at least 1.080 to give the foal optimal protection.

• The average foal nurses within 3 hours of birth. Some are slower than others and may require help. If your foal is three hours old and still hasn't mastered the art, give him 6 to 8 ounces of mare's colostrum from a baby bottle. Try to give the bottle in approximately the same position near the mare as he would be if he were nursing from her. If he still hasn't gotten the hang of it an hour later, try to help him learn by luring his lips to the mare's nipples with milk-coated fingers.

• Sometime within the first 12 hours after foaling, *no later*, give the mare a dose of ivermectin deworming paste.

CHAPTER 7

INDUCING LABOR

To induce or not to induce—this is one of those sharp controversies that seldom spawn much discussion—most horsepeople either believe it's "the only way to go" or they feel it's a terrible infringement of nature bordering on sacrilege. Any arguments against their point of view are either dismissed offhandedly or are simply not tolerated.

The truth is, when done properly, inducing labor in horses can be a real boon to the art and science of protecting mare and foal during the periparturient period. Nobody can argue with the fact that it's the only reliable way of ensuring that expert help is available when the foaling begins. It is also a great way of circumventing certain problems that can start small and evolve into something much larger if allowed to persist.

Unfortunately, however, when labor is induced solely for the sake of convenience, two important factors come into play. First, the "flavor" of the birthing scene becomes somewhat soured, as though an important natural event were now completely under the rigid control of man and his institutionalized medicine. Second, and definitely more importantly, when induction of labor becomes an accepted routine on a farm, the decision to induce often becomes a casual one, and the deadly serious guidelines regarding its safe implementation become faint and blurry or, worse, forgotten altogether.

A firm understanding of the physical and chemical events leading up to a *natural* birthing is mandatory if an intelligent decision about when to *induce* labor is to be made. Following are the most important considerations.

1. FOAL READINESS

Never forget that the mare gives birth in response to foal readiness rather than the numbers on a calendar. Don't let anyone convince you that "it's time" simply because the pregnancy is 340 days along, or because it's 328 days along and she foaled at 328 days last year. Every pregnancy is different, even if it appears externally identical to previous pregnancies.

Despite the fact that science knows a great deal about what triggers birthing in various species of animal (including man), very little is known about the horse in this regard. Since the best way to avoid problems in any medical procedure is to do it as closely as possible to the way it occurs naturally, the potential for problems in inducing labor in horses is higher than in most other species.

Most texts state that inducing labor is rational if the following three criteria are met: (1) the pregnancy is at least 320 days along, (2) the mare's milk is opaque white and (3) the cervix is soft. These clues are obviously changes in the *mare* that are interpreted to indicate the status of the *foal*, presuming that the mare has made these changes on the basis of communication she has received from the foal, telling her that *he* is ready.

Foal readiness means many things, including the foal's completed physical development. The last few weeks of pregnancy mark the period of time during which the foal makes the most profound progress in terms of increased size and weight, and in terms of the "finishing touches" associated with developmental maturity. Emerging from the uterus just a few days too soon may result in a foal that is too weak to stand and nurse, or a foal whose carpal ("knee") bones are still pliable due to incomplete calcification, and when he stands and subjects these bones to his body weight, they "smush" and leave him with permanently deformed legs. Or the foal may be unable to make all the important adaptations to life outside the uterus, and he dies at birth. The 320-day rule is not meant to suggest that the foal will always be adequately developed and likely to survive as long as he is at least 320 days along—the odds are certainly in his favor by that time, but there are no guarantees that his individual rate and style of development have placed him in the mainstream of "average-ness," and he may be a foal that requires 355 days to reach maximum survivability.

Foal readiness also relates to his position and his stage of preparation for the positional changes he will have to make in order to traverse the birth canal correctly. Remember that during Pre-Stage I, which encompasses two or three weeks prior to the actual birth, the foal is exercising the muscles and neuromuscular junctions of his neck and forelimbs, practicing and strengthening his ability to extend head and forelimbs into the birth canal so that they will be in this position when the mare rotates him over onto his side. This is one of the most crucial considerations of inducing labor—even if he is completely developed, **if labor is induced before the foal has had enough Pre-Stage I experience, he will surely be in the wrong position when the induced labor contractions begin**. In such a case, the foal's neck and/or forelimb(s) will be flexed in the abdomen, rather than extended (straightened) into the birth canal. This means two things with respect to inducing labor: first, be as certain as possible that it's not too early, and second, do not fail to check for foal position as soon as the water breaks, because the odds are increased that there will be a need for some remedial action.

Some authors have suggested that labor should not be induced unless the foal is in the "delivery position," but of course we all know now that in the normal situation the foal is not in the delivery position until he's already two-thirds of the way out of the mare. However, the foal does make a positional change that can be determined and used as a tool in deciding whether or not to induce. Prior to Pre-Stage I, the foal is almost always located way out of reach, in the abdomen. During Pre-Stage I, his head and forelimbs are often located in the birth canal, well within reach of an examiner's gloved and lubricated arm. Anybody who is trying to decide whether or not to induce labor in a mare should always include a proper palpation of the mare's vagina and cervix in the decision-making process. If all other factors have indicated that inducing labor is rational, the final factor should be the vaginal palpation—this will reveal whether or not the cervix is softened, and it will also show whether or not the foal is in the "extended" position, his head and forelimbs extended into the birth canal. If the foal is in this position, it is likely that he will be properly extended when the rotational contractions of early labor begin.

To perform the vaginal palpation, prepare the mare for the obstetrical procedure the same way as would be done if foal position were being checked during labor. Insert your gloved (sterile glove) and lubricated (sterile lube) hand into the mare's vagina in the proper manner, and gently and unobtrusively locate the cervix. It is important to be very gentle here, since you don't want to disturb the cervix. If the cervix is too tight to consider inducing labor, it will protrude into the vagina like a pointing finger. If this is what you find, your decision has been made, and there is no need to remain further in the vagina. If the cervix is soft, it may be difficult to find, since its lack of rigidity will make it somewhat indistinct to your exploring fingers. If the foal is already pushed partway through the cervix, labor has already officially begun.

After you have the information you need about the cervix, make an effort to determine where the foal is. In most cases, if he is in the extended position, he will be pushing at the wall of the vagina adjacent to the cervix, pushing that wall toward you with surprising force. The wall, fortunately, can be quite elastic, and it usually yields to the foal's pressure. The presence of your hand in the mare's vagina may appear to stimulate the foal to stretch and push even more. What you feel in a case like this is a hard protrusion, probably a leg or a muzzle or both, draped with the vaginal wall, so it may be difficult to identify exactly what part you're feeling, since you're feeling it through the vaginal wall.

2. MARE READINESS

Mare readiness is usually judged by the state of her udder, the character of the liquid it contains and the state of the cervix. Obviously the presence of adequate quantity and quality milk is essential for the maintenance of the foal once he is born, and the state of the cervix is important in ensuring that the foal will be able to squeeze through during the birthing process. More important, however, is the fact that specific hormonal events must take place in order for the milk and the cervix to be in the "delivery mode." Much of this hormonal "recipe" is still a mystery, but suffice it to say that as the foal achieves a certain level of development, specific signals are sent from his brain (the hypothalamus and pituitary, most likely) to the mare, and she responds to these signals by preparing her body for the delivery and the care of the foal after he is born.

In the context of inducing labor, all of this is important because it helps us to make an educated guess as to the foal's level of development. It is equally important, however, to bear in mind what we *don't* know about the natural birthing process in horses. For example, we don't know, specifically, what triggers it. We don't know whether the hormone prostaglandin, which is the predominant hormone present when the cervix is opening during the early stages of labor, is *causing* the cervix to open, or whether it is the *result* of the cervix opening. Why is this important? Well, it's important because prostaglandin is hormone #1 in a two-hormone process; in other words, **during the time when prostaglandin is the predominant hormone, rotational contractions of the uterus are taking place**. It's essential that these rotational contractions be allowed to progress to a certain point *before* expulsive contractions take place, because, as we discussed earlier in the book, if the uterus begins expelling the foal before he is adequately rotated, he will become jammed in the pelvic canal. Expulsive contractions are primarily due to hormone #2, oxytocin. Oxytocin is also the hormone that is most often used to induce labor. What happens if the "inducer" administers the oxytocin too early, before the mare's system has been adequately exposed to prostaglandin? Depending on the dose of oxytocin administered, it is probable that the oxytocin will cause expulsive contractions to occur abruptly, powerfully and prematurely, **before the uterus has had a chance to do any rotational contractions**. So, in a case like this, the mare will be pushing, valiantly, while the foal remains perfectly upside down. This is a serious problem, since the oxytocin has overridden the mare's ability to rotate the foal, and she will push and push until the foal is jammed.

Back to the vaginal palpation. One more clue that a mare

may give you if she is far enough along to justify inducing labor is the shedding of the cervical plug. Always check your glove after removing it from the mare—does it have a thick, sticky, pale pink–colored, pasty mucus on it? If so, she has already begun to shed the mucus plug that seals the cervix against contamination from the outside world. Shedding the mucus plug is one of the last things a mare does before going into labor, and if this has already begun to take place, your glove will pick up evidence of it while in the mare's vagina.

3. METHOD OF INDUCING LABOR

There are two main methods used in inducing labor when the survival of the foal is desired. The less popular of the two is the use of a prostaglandin injection. In theory, prostaglandin could be the more natural method, since we think it is one of the first hormones present during natural delivery. However, remember that we don't know whether the prostaglandin normally has a key role in the labor process or whether it is simply a side effect of the opening of the cervix. More importantly, prostaglandin is a much less reliable method of inducing labor. In some cases, delivery occurs a full 48 hours after the prostaglandin is given; in other cases it appears to take effect much sooner. In some cases it fails to work at all. Since one of the most rational reasons for inducing labor is to ensure that expert assistance will be on the scene when the mare goes into labor, it seems a little silly to use something that has such variable results.

There are documented cases of prostaglandin actually causing abortions in mares that are only in the first or second trimesters of pregnancy—it is well known that prostaglandin is a ubiquitous hormone that can be secreted by virtually every organ system in the body. If a pregnant mare breaks a leg, for example, the massive release of prostaglandin from the traumatized tissues at the fracture site may well lead to spontaneous abortion. Stress from a variety of sources, from scary thunderstorms to illness to long trailer rides, has been credited with causing prostaglandin release resulting in spontaneous abortions as well. Once again, however, individual horses seem to respond to the prostaglandin in their own way, some aborting the next day, some aborting the next week and some not aborting at all.

By far the more reliable and more popular method of inducing labor is by the injection of the hormone oxytocin. The injection almost always results in the birth of the foal within an hour. The fact that oxytocin *works* is not questioned—the salient point is that it takes careful thought and knowledge about the normal foaling to do an oxytocin induction without causing any harm. The most obvious way to cause harm is to do the induction too early in the course of the pregnancy, for reasons already discussed.

Another way to cause harm, however, is to administer an excessive dosage of oxytocin, or to administer it in a way that causes the onset of expulsive contractions too abruptly, too powerfully or too soon in the course of the labor process. If (and only if) it is intelligently determined that inducing labor is a rational decision, oxytocin should be given in a manner that introduces it into the mare's system gradually, allowing her body to do its preliminary work before the oxytocin's expulsive contractions get under way.

Oxytocin is generally available to veterinarians in a solution that is 20 international units (IU) per milliliter (ml). It can be given intramuscularly (IM) or intravenously (IV). If given IV, it can be given "straight" from the bottle, or diluted in a larger volume of sterile saline and given in a constant IV drip. An intramuscular injection takes a little time to be absorbed into the mare's bloodstream, so there is a natural delay in the onset of effect, and the result is a more gradual process that more closely mimics what happens in the normal, spontaneous delivery. An intravenous injection takes effect almost immediately, and the results can be quite violent, especially if the dosage is too high. Clinicians who prefer the IV route for some reason will avoid the abrupt, violent response by diluting the oxytocin in saline, thus giving the dosage over a longer period of time.

The proper dosage of oxytocin for inducing labor in a healthy mare carrying a mature pregnancy is 10 to 20 IU, which is only 0.5 to 1.0 ml or cc. Most oxytocin preparations indicate on the label that the proper dosage is up to 100 IU, or 5 ml—in my experience, a dosage this high is grossly unnecessary and borders on cruelty, and mares subjected to this kind of treatment may well turn themselves inside out in the process of giving birth. For inducing labor, the best procedure in my experience is the intramuscular injection of 20 IU (1 ml) of oxytocin. Approximately 20 minutes after the injection is given, the mare begins to sweat in the flank and underarm regions, in another 15 or 20 minutes she begins to raise her tail and pass frequent, small, moist manure piles, and before the hour is up, she breaks water and delivers her foal. For an induced foaling to occur any faster than this is to risk the onset of expulsive contractions before the foal has been adequately rotated and before the mare's cervix has had a chance to stretch widely enough to accommodate the emerging foal without being damaged. If the oxytocin is administered in this way and the mare appears not to respond at all after an hour, the decision to induce labor should definitely be reevaluated, since the mare's state of readiness should now be seriously in question.

BIBLIOGRAPHY

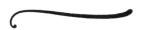

Adams, R., and Mayhew, I. Neurologic diseases. In Veterinary Clinics of North America, *Equine Practice*, vol. 1, no. 1 (April 1985): 209–234. Philadelphia: W. B. Saunders.

Asbury, A. C. Relationship of abnormality of the equine placenta to size, health, and vigor of the foal. In *Proceedings of the Annual Meeting of the Society for Theriogenology*, September 16–17, 1988: 306–10.

Baldwin, J. L., Vanderwall, D. K., Cooper, W. L., and Erb, H. N. Immunolobulin G and early survival of foals: a 3-year field study. In *Proceedings of the 35th Annual Convention of the American Association of Equine Practitioners*, Boston, Massachusetts, December 3–6, 1989: 179–86.

Becht, J. L., and Semrad, S. D. Gastrointestinal diseases of foals. In *The Compendium on Continuing Education*, vol. 8, no. 7: S367–73.

Blanchard, T. L. Managing the mare with hydroallantois. *Veterinary Medicine*, August 1989: 790–92.

Blanchard, T. L., et al. Management of dystocia in mares: examination, obstetrical equipment, and vaginal delivery. In *The Compendium on Continuing Education*, vol. 11, no 6 (June 1989): 745–753.

————. Equine Obstetrics: Mutation and delivery by traction. In *Theriogenology Handbook E-1* (3/89), Society for Theriogenology, American College of Theriogenologists: 1–4.

————. Uterine torsion in the mare. In *Theriogenology Handbook E-2* (3/89), Society for Theriogenology, American College of Theriogenologists: 1–3.

Bramlage, L. R., and Embertson R. M. Observations on the evaluation and selection of foal limb deformities for surgical treatment. In *Proceedings of the 36th Annual Convention of the American Association of Equine Practitioners*, December 2–5, 1990: 273–79.

Brewer, B. D. Pre- and immediate post-partum identification of the infected foal: the crucial role of the theriogenologist. In *Proceedings of the Annual Meeting of the Society for Theriogenology*, September 16–17, 1988: 322–27.

Clabough, D. L. Diseases of the equine neonate. *Equine Veterinary Science*, vol. 8, no. 1 (1988): 5–11.

Clarke, L. L., Roberts, M. C., and Argenzio, R. A. Feeding and digestive problems in horses: physiologic responses to a concentrated meal. In Veterinary Clinics of North America, *Equine Practice*, vol. 6, no. 2 (August 1990): 433–50. Philadelphia: W. B. Saunders.

Davis, L. E. Adverse drug reactions in the horse. In Veterinary Clinics of North America, *Equine Practice*, vol. 3, no. 1 (April 1987): 153–80. Philadelphia: W. B. Saunders.

DeBowes, R. M., Leipold, H. W., and Turner-Beatty, M. Cerebellar abiotrophy. In Veterinary Clinics of North America, *Equine Practice*, vol. 3, no. 2 (August 1987): 345–52. Philadelphia: W. B. Saunders.

Donoghue, S., Meacham, T. N., and Kronfeld, D. S. A conceptual approach to optimal nutrition of brood mares. In Veterinary Clinics of North America, *Equine Practice*, vol. 6, no. 2 (August 1990): 373–92. Philadelphia: W. B. Saunders.

Duren, S., Wood, C., and Jackson, S. Dietary fat and the racehorse. *Equine Veterinary Science*, vol. 7, no 6 (1987).

First, N. L., and Lohse, J. K. Mechanisms initiating and controlling parturition. In *Proceedings of the 10th International Congress on Animal Reproduction and Artificial Insemination*, Urbana-Champaign, Illinois, June 10–14, 1984: V31–42.

Ginther, O. J. *Reproductive Biology of the Mare*. Cross Plains, Wisconsin, Equiservices, 1979.

Ginther, O. J., and Adams, G. P. Equine fetal mobility as observed by video-imaging endoscopy. In *The Compendium on Continuing Education*, vol. 11, no. 10 (October 1989): 1275–80.

Haluska, G. J., and Wilkins, K. Predictive utility of pre-partum temperature changes in the mare. *Equine Veterinary Journal*, vol. 21, no. 2 (1989): 116–18.

Hawkins, K. L. Management of dystocia in the mare. In *Proceedings of the Annual Meeting of the Society for Theriogenology*, September 16–17, 1988: 69–72.

Hintz, H. Molds, mycotoxins, and mycotoxicosis. In Veterinary Clinics of North America, *Equine Practice*, vol. 6, no. 2 (August 1990): 419–32. Philadelphia: W. B. Saunders.

Houpt, K. A. Ingestive behavior. In Veterinary Clinics of North America, *Equine Practice*, vol. 6, no 2 (August 1990): 319–38. Philadelphia: W. B. Saunders.

Huston, R., Saperstein, G., and Leipold, H. W. Congenital defects in foals. *Journal of Equine Medicine and Surgery*, vol. 1, no. 4 (April 1977): 146–61.

Jones, W. E. Genetics and horse breeding. Philadelphia: Lea & Febiger, 1982.

Koterba, A. M. Effects of acute and chronic fetal hypoxia on the newborn. In *Proceedings of the Annual Meeting of the Society for Theriogenology*, September 16–17, 1988: 311–15.

———. Identification and early management of the high risk neonatal foal: averting disasters. *Equine Veterinary Education*, vol. 1, no. 1 (1989): 9–14.

Koterba, A. M., Drummond, W. H., and Kosch, P. Intensive care of the neonatal foal. In Veterinary Clinics of North America, *Equine Practice*, vol. 1, no. 1 (April 1985): 3–34. Philadelphia: W. B. Saunders.

———. Critical care of the neonatal foal. *Proceedings of a Satellite Video Conference*, Lenexa, Kansas: Veterinary Medicine Publishing Company, Inc., 1986.

Latimer, C. A., and Wyman, M. Neonatal ophthalmology. In Veterinary Clinics of North America, *Equine Practice*, vol. 1, no. 1 (April 1985): 235–60. Philadelphia: W. B. Saunders.

LeBlanc, M. H. Induction of parturition in the mare: significance of prepartum mammary secretions. In *Proceedings of the Annual Meeting of the Society for Theriogenology*, September 16–17, 1988: 85–88.

———. Update on passive transfer of immunoglobulins in foals, current modes of therapy. *Proceedings of the Annual Meeting of the Society for Theriogenology*, September 16–17, 1988: 316–21.

LeBlanc, M. H., et al. Epidural injection of xylazine for perineal analgesia in horses. *Journal of the American Veterinary Medical Association*, vol. 193, no. 11 (December 1988): 1405–1408.

Lewis, L. D. *Feeding and Care of the Horse*. Philadelphia: Lea & Febiger, 1982.

Ley, W. B., et al. Daytime foaling management of the mare 1: pre-foaling mammary secretions testing. *Equine Veterinary Science*, vol. 9, no. 2 (1989): 88–94.

———. Daytime foaling management of the mare 2: induction of parturition. *Equine Veterinary Science*, vol. 9, no. 2 (1989): 95–99.

Liu, I. K. M. Management and treatment of selected conditions in newborn foals. *Journal of the American Veterinary Medical Association*, vol. 176, no. 11 (June 1980): 1247–49.

———. Systemic diseases of the newborn foal. In Veterinary Clinics of North America, *Large Animal Practice*, vol. 2, no. 2 (November 1980): 361–75.

Madigan, J. E. Some practical aspects of feeding sick and convalescing foals. *Equine Practice*, September 1987: 924–28.

Mayhew, I., et al. Equine degenerative myeloencephalopathy: a vitamin E deficiency that may be familial. *Journal of Veterinary Internal Medicine*, vol. 1, no. 1: 45–50.

Monroe, J. L., et al. Effect of selenium and endophyte-contaminated fescue on performance and reproduction in mares. *Equine Veterinary Science*, vol. 8, no. 2 (1988): 148–52.

Mullaney, T. P., and Brown, C. M. Iron toxicity in neonatal foals. *Equine Veterinary Journal*, vol. 20, no. 2 (1988): 119–24.

National Academy of Sciences. *Atlas of Nutritional Data on U.S. and Canadian Feeds*, 1991.

O'Grady, S. E., and Roberts, L. A safe, simple way of bringing foals and "nurse mares" together. *Equine Practice*, July 1989: 719–20.

Pascoe, J. R., and Pascoe, R. R. Displacements, malpositions, and miscellaneous injuries of the mare's urogenital tract. In Veterinary Clinics of North America, *Equine Practice*, vol. 4, no. 3 (December 1988): 439–50. Philadelphia: W. B. Saunders.

Paul, J. W. Drug interactions and incompatibilities. In Veterinary Clinics of North America, *Equine Practice*, vol. 3, no. 1 (April 1987): 145–52. Philadelphia: W. B. Saunders.

Perry, J. S. The mammalian fetal membranes. *Journal of Reproductive Fertility*, vol. 62 (1981): 321–35.

Perryman, L. E., and McGuire, T. C. Evaluation for immune system failures in horses and ponies. *Journal of the American Veterinary Medical Association*, vol. 176, no. 12 (June 1980): 1374–77.

Prickett, M. E. Abortion and placental lesions in the mare. *Journal of the American Veterinary Medical Association*, vol. 157, no. 11 (1970): 1465–70.

Ralston, S. R., and Shideler, R. K. Inheritance of umbilical hernias in horses. In *Proceedings of the 10th International Congress on Animal Reproduction and Artificial Insemination*, Urbana-Champaign, Illinois, June 10–14, 1984: 530.

Randall, G. C. B. Perinatal adaptation. In *Proceedings of the 10th International Congress on Animal Reproduction and Artificial Insemination*, Urbana-Champaign, Illinois, June 10–14, 1984: V-43–50.

Reef, V. B. Cardiovascular disease in the equine neonate. In Veterinary Clinics of North America, *Equine Practice*, vol. 1, no. 1 (April 1985): 117–29. Philadelphia: W. B. Saunders.

Roberts, S. J. Veterinary Obstetrics and Genital Diseases. 3rd Ed. Woodstock, Vermont, S. J. Roberts: 1986.

Robertson, J. T., and Embertson, R. M. Surgical management of congenital and perinatal abnormalities of the urogenital tract. In Veterinary Clinics of North America, *Equine Practice*, vol. 4, no. 3 (December 1988): 359–80. Philadelphia: W. B. Saunders.

Rooney, J. R., Sack, W. O., and Habel R. E. *Guide to the Dis-*

section of the Horse. Ithaca, New York: Wolfgang O. Sack, 1967.

Rossdale, P. D., and Ricketts, S. W. Equine stud farm medicine. 2nd ed. Philadelphia: Lea & Febiger, 1980.

Schuijt, G. Iatrogenic fractures of ribs and vertebrae during delivery in perinatally dying calves: 235 cases (1978–1988). *Journal of the American Veterinary Medical Association,* vol. 197, no. 9 (November 1, 1990): 1196–1202.

Slone, D. E. Ovariectomy, ovariohysterectomy, and cesarean section in mares. In Veterinary Clinics of North America, *Equine Practice,* vol. 4, no. 3 (December 1988): 451–60. Philadelphia: W. B. Saunders.

Swerczek, T. W. Pathology and pathogenesis of equine fetal disease. In *Proceedings of the Annual Meeting of the Society for Theriogenology,* 1976: 46–55.

——. Equine fetal diseases. In *Current Veterinary Therapy in Theriogenology,* 2nd ed., David A. Morrow, ed. 699–704. Philadelphia: W. B. Saunders, 1986.

Taylor, T. S., et al. Management of dystocia in mares: uterine torsion and cesarean section. In *The Compendium on Continuing Education,* vol. 11, no. 10 (October 1989): 1265–72.

United States National Research Council (NRC). *Nutrient Requirements of Horses,* 5th rev. ed., Washington, D.C.: National Academy Press, 1989.

Vandeplassche, M., and Lauwers, H. The twisted umbilical cord: an expression of kinesis of the equine fetus? *Animal Reproduction Science,* vol. 10 (1986): 163–75.

Veterinary Report. Study shows worming mares has effect on foals. University of Illinois, Spring 1989.

Villahoz, M. D., et al. Reproductive problems of pregnant mares grazing fescue pastures in Argentina. In *Proceedings of the 10th International Congress on Animal Reproduction and Artificial Insemination,* Urbana-Champaign, Illinois, June 10–14, 1984: 100.

Waelchli, R. O., et al. Relationships of total protein, specific gravity, viscosity, refractive index and latex agglutination to immunoglobulin G concentration in mare colostrum. *Equine Veterinary Journal,* vol. 22, no. 1 (1990): 39–42.

Wagner, P. C., Grant, B. D., and Reed S. M. Cervical vertebral malformations. In Veterinary Clinics of North America,

Equine Practice, vol. 3, no. 2 (August 1987): 385–96. Philadelphia: W. B. Saunders.

Wagner, P. C., and Watrous, B. J. Equine pediatric orthopedics: part 3—tendon laxity and rupture. *Equine Practice*, vol. 12, no. 6 (June 1990): 19–22.

Whitwell, K. E. Infective placentitis in the mare. In *Proceedings of the 5th International Conference on Equine Infectious Diseases*, 1987: 172–80.

Witherspoon, D. M. Some reflections concerning Caslick's surgery, ultrasonography and the treatment of uterine cysts. *Equine Practice*, vol. 11, no. 9 (September 1989): 12–15. Philadelphia: W. B. Saunders.

Youngquist, R. S. Equine referral hospital dystocias. In *Proceedings of the Annual Meeting of the Society for Theriogenology*, September 16–17, 1988: 73–84.

INDEX

THE SATURDAY BIG TENT WEDDING PARTY

THE SATURDAY BIG TENT
WEDDING PARTY

Alexander McCall Smith

Alfred A. Knopf Canada

PUBLISHED BY ALFRED A. KNOPF CANADA

Copyright © 2011 Alexander McCall Smith

www.randomhouse.ca

Library and Archives Canada Cataloguing in Publication

McCall Smith, Alexander, 1948–
The Saturday big tent wedding party / Alexander McCall Smith.

(No. 1 Ladies' Detective Agency series)
Issued also in an electronic format.

ISBN 978-0-307-39826-0

I. Title. II. Series: McCall Smith, Alexander, 1948– . No. 1 Ladies'
Detective Agency series.

PR6063.C326S37 2011   823'.914   C2010-904223-9

First Edition

Printed and bound in the United States of America

2 4 6 8 9 7 5 3 1

This book is for Professor Max Essex
of the Harvard AIDS Initiative,
in admiration of the work that he has done.

THE SATURDAY BIG TENT WEDDING PARTY

THE MEMORY OF LOST THINGS

MA RAMOTSWE had by no means forgotten her late white van. It was true that she did not brood upon it, as some people dwell on things of the past, but it still came to mind from time to time, often at unexpected moments. Memories of that which we have lost are curious things—weeks, months, even years may pass without any recollection of them and then, quite suddenly, something will remind us of a lost friend, or of a favourite possession that has been mislaid or destroyed, and then we will think: *Yes, that is what I had and I have no longer.*

Her van had been her companion and friend for many years. Can a vehicle—a collection of mechanical bits and pieces, nuts and bolts and parts the names of which one has not the faintest idea of—can such a thing be a friend? Of course it can: physical objects can have personalities, at least in the eyes of their owners. To others, it may only be a van, but to the owner it may be the friend that has started loyally each morning—except sometimes; that has sat patiently during long hours of waiting outside the houses of suspected adulterers; that has carried one home in the late afternoon, tired after a day's work at the No. 1 Ladies' Detective Agency. And just like a person, a car or a van may have likes and dislikes. A good tar road is balm to man and machine and may produce a humming sound of satisfaction in both car and driver; an unpaved road, concealing behind each bend a deep pothole or tiny mountain range of corrugations, may provoke rattles and groans of protest from even the most tolerant of vehicles. For this reason, the owners of cars may be forgiven for thinking that under the metal there lurks something not all that different from a human soul.

Mma Ramotswe's van had served her well, and she loved it. Its life, though, had been a hard one. Not only had it been obliged to cope with dust, which, as anybody who lives in a dry country will know, can choke a vehicle to death, but its long-suffering suspension had been required to deal with persistent overloading, at least on the driver's side. That, of course, was the side on which Mma Ramotswe sat, and she was, by her own admission and description, a traditionally built person. Such a person can wear down even the toughest suspension, and this is exactly what happened in the case of the tiny white van, which permanently listed to starboard as a result.

Mma Ramotswe's husband, Mr. J.L.B. Matekoni, that excellent man, proprietor of Tlokweng Road Speedy Motors and widely regarded as the best mechanic in all Botswana, had done his best to address the problem, but had tired of having to change the van's shock absorbers from side to side so as to equalise the strain. Yet it went further than that. The engine itself had started to make a sinister sound, which grew in volume until eventually the big-end failed.

"I am just a mechanic, Mma Ramotswe," he had said to his wife. "A mechanic is a man who fixes cars and other vehicles. That is what a mechanic does."

Mma Ramotswe had listened politely, but her heart within her was a stone of fear. She knew that the fate of her van was at